U0292183

肿瘤研究

前沿

第16卷

樊代明 主编

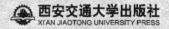
西安交通大学出版社
XI'AN JIAOTONG UNIVERSITY PRESS

内容简介

本书是全面介绍肿瘤研究进展的系列著作——《肿瘤研究前沿》的第16卷。全书共分为七章，介绍肿瘤研究领域的最新进展，反映的内容都是当前肿瘤研究的热点和前沿。本书可作为相关专业研究人员的参考用书，也可供高校、医院的相关人员阅读使用。

图书在版编目（CIP）数据

肿瘤研究前沿. 第16卷/樊代明主编. —西安:西安交通大学出版社,2016.11
ISBN 978 - 7 - 5605 - 9005 - 9

Ⅰ.①肿… Ⅱ.①樊… Ⅲ.①肿瘤—研究 Ⅳ.①R73

中国版本图书馆 CIP 数据核字（2016）第 221701 号

书　　名	肿瘤研究前沿（第16卷）
主　　编	樊代明
责任编辑	宋伟丽　黄　璐
出版发行	西安交通大学出版社
	（西安市兴庆南路10号　邮政编码710049）
网　　址	http://www.xjtupress.com
电　　话	（029）82668357　82667874（发行中心）
	（029）82668315（总编办）
传　　真	（029）82668280
印　　刷	虎彩印艺股份有限公司
开　　本	850mm×1168mm　1/32　印张　7.75　字数　178千字
版次印次	2016年11月第1版　2016年11月第1次印刷
书　　号	ISBN 978 - 7 - 5605 - 9005 - 9/R·1399
定　　价	62.00元

读者购书、书店添货,如发现印装质量问题,请与本社发行中心联系、调换。
订购热线:(029)82665248　(029)82665249
投稿热线:(029)82668803　(029)82668804
读者信箱:med_xjup@163.com

版权所有　侵权必究

编委会

主　　编：樊代明

编　　者：（按姓氏拼音排序）

樊代明　郭　阳　韩　宇　洪　流

李　铤　李进晶　刘　刚　柳金强

马娇娇　聂勇战　时永全　帖　君

王　颖　温伟红　吴　键　吴介恒

张　磊　张向远　周　威

学术秘书：杨志平

主 编 简 介

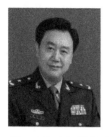

樊代明,消化病学专家,重庆人。现任中国工程院副院长(党组成员)、第四军医大学西京消化病医院院长、肿瘤生物学国家重点实验室主任、国家药物临床试验机构主任、中国抗癌协会副理事长、亚太消化学会副主席,曾任第四军医大学校长、中华消化学会主任委员、2013年世界消化病大会主席,首批国家杰出青年基金和首批长江学者特聘教授获得者。

长期从事消化系疾病的临床与基础研究工作,并致力于医学发展的宏观战略研究,在国际上率先提出整合医学的理论与实践。先后承担国家"973"首席科学家项目、"863"项目、攻关项目、重大新药创制、自然科学基金、工程院重大咨询项目等课题。获国家科技进步一、二、三等奖各1项,国家技术发明奖1项,军队科技进步一等奖2项,陕西省科学技术一等奖2项,国家发明专利38项、实用新型专利16项,国家新药证书1项。获美国国家医学院外籍院士、法国国家医学院塞维亚奖、何梁何利科技进步奖、陕西省科技最高成就奖、求是实用工程奖等多项荣誉奖励。主编专著21本,其中《精——樊代明院士治学之道》和《医学发展考》两本均为长达210余万字、厚近1500页的大型著作。担任"临床基础医学精读系列"丛书(10 册)和《肿瘤研究前沿》(16 册)的总主编,还是"全国高等教育医学数字化规划教材"(53 册)的总主编。担任 *Nature Reviews Gastroenterology & Hepatology*、*Gut* 等 10 本国际杂志的编委、副主编或主编。在 *Lancet*、*Nature Reviews Gastroenterology & Hepatology*、*Nature Clinical Practice Oncology*、*Gut* 等国外杂志发表 SCI 论文 583 篇,单篇最高影响因子 45 分,论文被引用逾 1 万次。培养研究生共 173 名,其中获全国优秀博士论文 5 名,获全军优秀博士论文 10 名。

2001 年当选中国工程院院士。

序

　　肿瘤是严重危害人类健康及生命的疾病。尽管国内外已投入大量的人力和财力进行研究,发表的论著也有成千上万,但至今对其病因和发病机制尚不清楚,多数肿瘤在临床诊断、治疗及预防方面也无重大突破。造成这种现状的根本原因除了肿瘤本身的复杂性外,还与各专业的研究者之间沟通较少、"各行其是",对肿瘤研究的全貌及进展了解不够、顾此失彼,以及各专业在理论及技术上的协作欠佳有关。要解决这个问题,需要有人把各专业对肿瘤研究的重大进展及时进行整理总结并加以评述,从中找出相互间研究的生长点及解决办法,然后适时地介绍给正在或将要从事肿瘤研究的同事。《肿瘤研究前沿》将会适应这种需求,结合著者自己的科研成果,将目前世界上肿瘤研究的最新进展尽力以最通俗的语言介绍给同行及相关研究人员,每年一卷,各卷介绍的内容有所侧重,连续下去,坚持数年,必有好处。如无特殊情况,直至肿瘤被攻克之日。

　　本书像专著,因为它含有著者的研究成果;它像综述,因为它介绍世界文献的最新进展;它像述评,因为它给出著者的观点及见解;它也像科普读物,因为它力求以最普通的文字面对读者。它以包容性、先进性、焦点争论为特色。这就是它既像什么又不完全是什么的缘故,这就是肿瘤研究的现状,也就是本书追逐的肿瘤研究的前沿。

樊代明

2001.8

目　　录

第一章

CypB/STAT3/miR-520d-5p 环路在胃癌炎癌转化过程中的作用机制

　　胃癌是世界范围内致死率第二的恶性肿瘤，而70%的新发病例和死亡病例出现在包括我国在内的发展中国家。因此研究胃癌的发生、发展机制对于我国预防胃癌发生、遏制胃癌进展以及降低胃癌的死亡率具有重要指导意义。

　　胃癌的发生被广泛认为同幽门螺旋杆菌（helicobacter pylori，Hp）感染及继发的炎症反应有密切关系。自从1984年发现Hp感染是造成胃和十二指肠溃疡以及慢性胃炎以来，多项研究陆续证明Hp感染能使胃癌发生率明显上升。通过促进包括白细胞介素6（interleukin 6，IL-6）、白细胞介素8（interleukin 8，IL-8）在内的多种炎症因子释放，Hp在胃癌的发生、增殖、转移等发展过程中发挥了重要作用。总的来说，IL-6激活的STAT3在胃肠道上皮细胞的恶性转化中扮演了关键的角色。作为多条癌基因通路的交汇点，STAT3（信号转导及转录激活因子3）的激活被发现能促进多种肿瘤的增殖、存活、血管生成以及转移，并能够抑制抗肿瘤免疫。STAT3在多种肿瘤中均被发现为持续激活状态，且其激活是维持肿瘤增殖和抑制凋亡状态的必要条件。但是，STAT3在肿瘤细胞中被持续激活的原因尚未完全阐明。

　　IL-6刺激能造成STAT3的磷酸化并向细胞核转移，同特定的DNA序列结合，从而调控STAT3下游分子的转录。近期研究发现，STAT3被激活的过程同亲环素B（cyclophillin B，CypB）

的表达失常有关。CypB 属于亲环素家族，是环孢素 A 的细胞内受体，其肽酰脯氨酰异构酶活性在蛋白质折叠过程中有重要作用。CypB 主要定位于细胞的内质网中，其在肝炎病毒复制、免疫抑制、催乳素信号通路转导以及骨质疏松发生等机体生理或病理过程中发挥重要作用。研究者发现在黑色素瘤和恶性胶质瘤中，CypB 的存在对于 STAT3 的激活有不可或缺的作用。敲除或药物抑制 CypB 导致 JAK/STAT3 通路的抑制及细胞死亡。此外，CypB 被发现在包括黑色素瘤、肝癌、胰腺癌、恶性胶质瘤及乳腺癌等在内的多种肿瘤中过表达，但是 CypB 在肿瘤中过表达的机制及其同 STAT3 的关系尚不明确。

　　MicroRNA（miRNA，微小 RNA）是一类长度为 20 ~ 22 nt 的小 RNA（核糖核酸），通过结合靶基因信使的非翻译区导致其翻译抑制或直接降解。我们前期的生物信息学分析结果显示 miR - 520d - 5p 在 CypB 的 3′端非翻译区具有潜在结合位点，且二者表达水平在胃癌细胞和组织中均负相关。近期几项研究也指出 miR - 520 家族的 miRNA 在多种肿瘤中具有抑癌作用。综合以上文献及我们的初步研究结果，我们建立了 miR - 520d - 5p 可能是 CypB 的上游调控分子的假说。另外，有研究证实了 STAT3 通过直接结合相应分子的启动子区域发挥对多个 miRNA 的靶向调控作用。miRNA 经常同其靶分子形成反馈通路。这是因为调控它们的转录因子同时也可能是它们本身的直接或间接的靶分子。这些调控环路是肿瘤相关信号通路的核心，因为它们在细胞受到炎症因素影响下由正常向肿瘤转变过程中帮助促进并维持细胞表型的持续变化。因此 miR - 520d - 5p 作为 CypB 的调控分子将 CypB 同 STAT3 的激活以及胃癌的炎症 - 肿瘤转化联系在了一起。

　　本文中我们提供了一系列证据显示一条由 IL - 6 诱导的 CypB/STAT3/miR - 520d - 5p 反馈通路在胃癌发展过程中的促进

作用。我们研究发现 CypB 的过表达是 STAT3 在胃癌中激活的必要条件；随后我们证实 miR-520d-5p 在转录水平直接抑制 CypB 的表达；此外，miR-520d-5p 也是 STAT3 的调控基因。这条反馈通路的发现，有助于理解幽门螺旋杆菌感染和炎症反应造成 IL-6 分泌促进胃癌中 STAT3 持续激活的原因，并为治疗胃癌恶性进展提供新的思路。

一、Hp 通过炎症导致胃癌

（一）胃癌和 Hp 感染

胃癌是世界范围内肿瘤导致死亡的第二大原因。幽门螺旋杆菌感染是导致胃癌的最重要的危险因素。目前估测全球约有 50% 的人口感染该病原体，它导致了胃炎、消化性溃疡、胃癌以及黏膜相关的淋巴组织淋巴瘤。由于 75% 的胃癌归因于 Hp 感染，世界卫生组织已经将它划分为一类致癌物。

胃癌发生的危险因素包括 CagA 阳性的 Hp 感染、Hp 的系统地理学起源以及包括 IL-1、IL-8、IL-10、TNF-α 和 IFN-γ 在内的基因多态性。在 Hp 感染后，宿主的免疫系统会被诱发非特异和特异性免疫应答，并产生多种激素反应。而除了如此激烈的炎症反应外，除持续使用抗生素外很难达到病原体的清除，这也导致了终身感染和继发的炎症。慢性炎症进而导致组织损伤、氧化应激和 DNA（脱氧核糖核酸）损伤。我们推测这些感染造成的不良反应为胃黏膜创造了促癌的微环境并促进胃上皮细胞恶性转化。因此，探索 Hp 感染造成的慢性炎症的本质及其导致胃癌发生的原因是非常有必要的。

（二）Hp 的毒力

近期的证据显示 Hp 导致的慢性炎症和氧化应激为细胞的 DNA 损伤和组织损伤创造微环境。DNA 损伤导致基因不稳定性并最终导致恶性转化。病原体编码的蛋白等致病因素诱导了稳定的免疫激活并改变了宿主的基因信号通路，降低了癌变的阈值，包括 DNA 损伤修复、聚胺合成和分解、抗氧化反应以及细胞因子合成。

1. CagA 同胃癌发生的关系

CagA 是 Hp 的毒力因素中最为重要的一员，对胃黏膜上皮细胞和免疫细胞有多重影响。同 CagA 阴性 Hp 感染的个体相比，感染 CagA 阳性 Hp 的个体发生胃癌的危险度上升明显。CagA 蛋白通过 T4SS 蛋白复合体被转入宿主细胞，后者同 CagA 基因位点接近。一旦进入细胞，宿主细胞的蛋白激酶会磷酸化 CagA，从而启动了 CagA 的一系列功能的发挥（图 1 - 1），包括 MAPK（丝裂原活化蛋白激酶）信号通路的激活，凋亡信号通路的抑制，细胞生长的阻滞以及细胞运动的失调。CagA 阳性的 Hp 被发现能在胃黏膜上皮细胞诱导更高水平的 TNF - α、IL - 1β 及 IL - 8，这些细胞因子都是炎症因子且能够诱导活性氧物质（reactive oxygen species，ROS）的发生。此外，近期一项研究发现 CagA 阳性 Hp 感染能够显著增加细胞 H_2O_2 的产生。结果，感染的细胞和胃组织出现了 DNA 损伤和突变的增加——尤其在癌基因和抑癌基因位置——这些是肿瘤发生的重要分子基础。因此，这些结果提示 CagA 诱导的 DNA 损伤是感染和胃癌发生之间的联系的关键。

2. VacA 同胃癌发生的关系

另一个 Hp 同胃癌发生相关的毒力因素是 VacA，其能够增加 Hp 定植在胃黏膜的成功率。另外，VacA s1m1 等位基因阳性的菌株被发现同慢性胃炎严重程度和癌症发生危险性相关。但是 VacA 导致这些变化的机制尚不清楚。

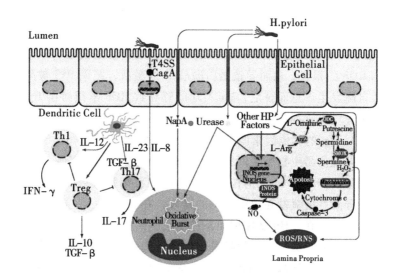

图 1-1　胃黏膜中 Hp 同免疫细胞的联系

Hp 感染导致 IL-8 产生，这种 IL-8 产生依赖于 CagA。IL-8 募集了中性粒细胞，Hp 的 NapA 和尿激酶导致中性粒细胞的氧化反应，使其产生大量的 ROS 并分泌入感染的微环境中。此外，NapA 能够促进中性粒细胞存活，从而进一步促进了氧化应激反应的进行。感染还能够诱导巨噬细胞产生 iNOS，导致一氧化氮产生。同时，感染造成树突状细胞分泌细胞因子的改变，向调节性 T 细胞方向倾斜（引自 J Leuk Biol, 2014, 96: 201-212）

　　线粒体膜是 VacA 的靶点之一。一项研究通过 DCFDA 染色发现，VacA 导致细胞膜的 ROS 产生明显增多。这些反应同样在嗜酸性粒细胞和 Hela 细胞中被发现。同时，VacA 导致了钙离子的释放并进而激活了 NF-κB 信号通路。激活的 NF-κB 通路活性导致炎症因子的释放，进一步募集免疫细胞到达感染部位。

VacA被发现同时具有促进和抑制细胞自噬的功能。近期一项研究发现VacA在胃上皮细胞中能够干扰自噬的发生。自噬是清除包括ROS在内的细胞内成分的关键生理过程。因此VacA介导的自噬阻断导致细胞内ROS的聚集。而与此相反，另一项研究发现VacA能够诱导上皮细胞的自噬。VacA能够同LRP1（低密度脂蛋白受体相关蛋白1）结合，而后者的激活导致细胞内ROS的积聚，从而导致蛋白激酶B的激活，结果P53被降解而自噬发生。总而言之，VacA均能够导致ROS累积而在Hp感染过程中促进细胞氧化应激。

3. Hp的其他因素同胃癌发生的关系

其他的微生物因素同样能够被Hp感染诱导并在炎症反应中发挥重要作用。NapA的作用主要是中性粒细胞向感染部位的募集，导致自由氧基在感染部位的释放。有趣的是，由于NapA依赖的机制存在，Hp受保护而不被氧化基团损伤。

尿激酶是另一个能够招募中性粒细胞到感染部位的Hp毒力因子。重组尿激酶足够诱导小鼠模型的中性粒细胞的浸润，进而导致ROS水平升高和炎症反应加剧。一般而言是寿命较短的，但这些浸润的中性粒细胞对凋亡耐受，故有较长寿命因而对机体有害。另外，尿激酶能够激活巨噬细胞产生iNOS（诱导型一氧化氮合酶），因而促进固有免疫应答并加重炎症反应。

Hp的伽玛谷氨酰转移酶（gamma-glutamyl transpeptidese，GGT）能够刺激胃上皮细胞产生H_2O_2从而加重疾病。这些反应诱导NF-κB的激活和IL-8的产生。IL-8是炎症诱导因子，在Hp感染的胃上皮组织中高表达，其通过招募中性粒细胞来介导炎症反应。此外，IL-8还有促癌作用。研究者将rGGT加入到胃上皮细胞中后，通过流式细胞仪检测细胞DNA损伤的指示剂8-OHdG明显增高。上调的ROS、炎症介导因子，以及DNA氧化损伤为胃上皮细胞的恶性转化创造了理想条件。

（三）Hp 通过 IL－6 影响胃癌发生

Hp 感染导致慢性胃炎过程中，IL－6 的产生及其下游信号通路的激活在胃癌的发生中起了关键作用。不少研究发现，Hp 的感染能够显著促进胃黏膜中 IL－6 的产生。一项在蒙古沙鼠模型中的研究发现，感染野生型 Hp 48 周后，沙鼠胃黏膜细胞的 IL－6 的 mRNA 水平明显升高，在 12 个月后达到最高峰，这种变化可能是由 Hp 的膜表面蛋白诱导出现的。一项针对 Hp 感染的日本成人的调查研究发现，受检人群血清中的 IL－6 水平同 Hp 的抗体水平明显正相关。这提示 Hp 的感染可能促进 IL－6 的产生。还有研究发现，Hp 感染的患者胃黏膜中 IL－6 的水平明显高于 Hp 阴性的胃炎患者。这提示 IL－6 在 Hp 相关的胃炎疾病进展中的潜在病理作用。

Hp 被发现通过 IL－6 受体激活 STAT3 信号通路。研究者发现，感染 Hp 的胃上皮细胞的 STAT3 磷酸化水平升高，并出现从细胞质到细胞核的定位转位现象。荧光素酶实验也证实 STAT3 信号通路被激活。进一步研究发现 STAT3 的激活是依赖于 CagA 蛋白的进入细胞而非磷酸化。研究结果表明，STAT3 的激活是通过 IL－6 受体实现的，并能够被 gp130 抗体导致的 gp130 抑制所诱发。但是，这种激活同 IL－6 或者 IL－11 的自分泌无明显关系。总之，这些结果证实 Hp 能够通过 CagA 蛋白在体内和体外激活 STAT3 信号通路。

IL－6 是被研究最为深入的促癌细胞因子之一。它的家族中包括 IL－11、IL－27、IL－31、白血病抑制因子（leukemia inhibitory factor，LIF）、OSM（抑瘤素 M）、CNTF（睫状神经营养因子）、CT－1 以及心肌营养素样因子（cardiotrophin-like cytokirl，CLC）等。这些细胞因子能够影响细胞增殖、存活、分化、迁移、侵袭、转移、血管生成、炎症以及代谢（图 1 - 2）。
IL - 6 家族成员中除 IL - 31 之外，均能够通过特定受体和共同
的受体亚单位 gp130 激活 JAK - STAT3 信号通路、PI3K - AKT
通路和 MAPK - ERK 通路。在这些通路中，STAT3 是 gp130 的主
要下游信号通路，它是连接炎症和肿瘤发生的癌基因。在既往
的研究中，IL - 6 被发现在包括皮肤癌、乳腺癌、肺癌、食管
癌、肾癌、肝癌、胰腺癌、胃癌、结肠癌、卵巢癌、前列腺癌、
膀胱癌、血液系统肿瘤及黑色素瘤在内的多种肿瘤中表达升高，
这表明 IL - 6 可能在癌症发生过程中具有非常重要的作用。因而
研究 IL - 6/STAT3 信号通路在胃癌中的作用机制对于理解肿瘤
恶性表型的分子基础至关重要。

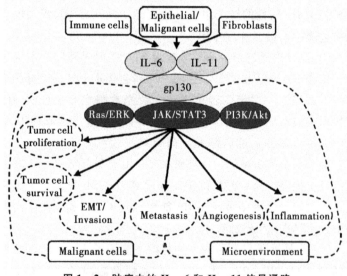

图 1 - 2 肿瘤中的 IL - 6 和 IL - 11 信号通路

免疫细胞、成纤维细胞以及上皮细胞产生 IL - 6 和 IL - 11 能够激活 JAK - STAT3、
SHP - 2 - RAS - ERK 通路和 PI3K - AKT 通路，进而促进细胞增殖、存活、EMT、侵
袭、转移、血管生成和炎症反应（引自 Semin Immunol，2014，26：54 - 74）

1. IL－6 信号通路传导机制

IL－6 能够同细胞膜表面的 IL－6 受体 α 结合，形成复合体并同 gp130 形成二聚体（图 1－3）。此外，生理情况下细胞中存在可溶性的 IL－6 受体和 gp130，这些分子由细胞内的酶将膜上的 IL－6 受体特异性剪切产生。分泌性的 IL－6 受体在不依赖膜 IL－6 受体情况下也能够激活 gp130。这种机制可能是介导炎症促进反应发生的主要机制，而经典的膜 IL－6 受体可能介导了炎症抑制反应的发生。Gp130 同 IL－6/IL－6 受体复合物结合后，三种主要的信号通路能够被激活。第一种是 JAK－STAT 信号通路。结合造成了 gp130 的二聚化，招募了相关的 JAK 磷酸化激酶（JAK1、JAK2 和 Tyk2）靠近并促使它们发生相互磷酸化和激活。JAK 激酶磷酸化 gp130 在细胞质内的酪氨酸位点，因而创造了能够提供 STAT 蛋白、SHP－2 蛋白和 SOCS3 蛋白的 SH2 结构域结合的位点。结果，JAK 激酶直接磷酸化了 STAT3 和 STAT1，而激活的 STAT 蛋白形成了二聚体并进入细胞核发挥转录作用。Gp130 的二聚化显著激活 STAT3，也相对较弱激活 STAT1。IL－6 诱导的 STAT3 激活能被 SOCS3 快速抑制，后者是 STAT3 的靶基因所编码的蛋白。SOCS3 抑制 STAT3 激活的机制是其能够同时结合 JAK 和 gp130 并直接覆盖 JAK1、JAK2 和 TYK2 的催化结构域。激活的 STAT3 蛋白抑制剂（protein inhibitor of activated STAT3，PIAS3）也被报道是 STAT3 的内源性抑制剂，其通过结合 STAT3 二聚体发挥作用。但近期一项研究发现近期一项研究发现，STAT3 的持续激活可能和 IL－6 受体同 EGFR 的联系有关，这种结合对 STAT3 的激活能够逃逸 SOCS3 的抑制，因为 EGFR 不能被 SOCS3 识别。这种激活的信号通路能够导致强烈的癌基因激活效应。第二种信号通路是 SHP－2/Ras/ERK 信号通路。SHP－2 的募集通过 JAK 激酶和 Gab1 结合导致自身的磷酸化，这是该信号通路的启动反应。最后一种

gp130 信号通路是 PI3K – AKT 通路，这条通路的激活机制尚不明确，但可能同 SHP – 2 和 Gab1 有关。

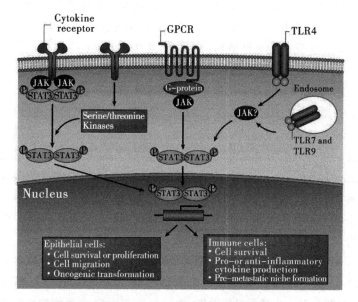

图 1 – 3　肿瘤中 JAK – STAT3 通路的激活机制

（引自 Nat Rev Cancer, 2014, 14：736 – 746）

2. IL – 6 和细胞增殖、存活、分化

IL – 6 通过多条信号通路对肿瘤细胞的生长发挥促进作用。除细胞增殖和存活外，IL – 6 – STAT3 分子通路还调控 Th17 细胞、巨噬细胞以及树突状细胞的分化。IL – 6 上调造成的 STAT3 激活能够上调 Cyclin D1、D2 和 B1，以及 c – Myc，并抑制 Cdk 抑制分子 P21 的表达，因而促进细胞进入细胞周期循环。IL – 6 也是细胞存活的重要调控分子，能够帮助肿瘤细胞逃逸应急和化疗药物造成的细胞死亡。IL – 6 激活的 STAT3 能够促进存活相关蛋白的表达，包括 Bcl – 2、Bcl – XL、Mcl – 1、Survivin 和

XIAP。这些蛋白的上调和持续激活的 STAT3 通常同肿瘤化疗耐药的机制有关。另外，IL-6 通过增加端粒酶活性抑制细胞衰老，从而促进细胞生长。IL-6 也能够通过介导 EGF（表皮生长因子）和 HGF（肝细胞生长因子）家族的相互作用来促进增殖。IL-11 也通过类似的机制促进细胞增殖，抑制细胞凋亡。

3. IL-6 通路同 microRNA

　　MicroRNA 是一种重要的调控基因表达的内源性调控机制，其表达在多种肿瘤细胞中均有明显的变化。miRNA 同样在炎症-肿瘤转化过程中发挥重要的调控作用。细胞因子能够调控 miRNA 的转录和表达，而 miRNA 也能够反过来调控细胞因子的信号通路相关蛋白的表达。近期研究发现 miRNA 在 IL-6 介导的细胞存活和 IL-6 通路的调控中占重要角色（图 1-4）。miR-21 被认为是在多种肿瘤细胞中高表达的癌基因。它在肿瘤发生和转移中的功能可能同其靶基因 PTEN、Spry1 等抑癌基因有关。miR-21 在恶性骨髓瘤和胆管细胞癌等高表达 IL-6 的肿瘤中均表达异常升高。进一步研究发现 IL-6 刺激后，STAT3 被募集到 miR-21 的启动子区域并促进 miR-21 的转录本的表达。miR-21 还在 IL-11-STAT3 通路的抑制凋亡通路中发挥关键作用。另外，在胆管癌细胞中过表达 IL-6 后可发现 let-7 的表达升高，而其靶基因 NF2 的表达受到抑制。相反，let-7 的表达水平降低被发现在肺癌、Burkit 淋巴瘤和乳腺癌中是癌基因 NF-κB 激活导致的 LIN-28B 这种 let-7 的抑制因子升高的结果。有趣的是，let-7a 能够直接靶向抑制 IL-6 本身，因而 LIN28B 导致的 let-7 降低能够引起 IL-6 表达的升高，进而促进细胞恶性转化。IL-6 还能够通过促进 miR-17/92 簇的表达进而促进自身信号通路的转导。SOCS1 是 IL-6-STAT3 信号通路的抑制剂，近期研究发现其也是 miR-17/92 家族 miRNA 的靶分子。因此，在骨髓瘤的细胞系中抑制 miR-17/92 的表达后，SOCS1 的表达被上调，而 STAT3 的磷酸化水平被显著抑制。miR－204、miR－211 和 miR－379 在乳腺癌细胞中能够直接靶向 IL－11 的 mRNA 发挥调控作用；另外，不少 miRNA 也能够调控 IL－6 通路：miR－26a 通过抑制 IL－6 的表达抑制肝癌细胞生长和转移，miR－146a 在小鼠巨噬细胞中通过抑制 Notch1 信号通路抑制 IL－6 的产生，miR－30c 通过抑制 IL－11 的表达抑制乳腺癌细胞的化疗耐受，miR－19a 能够促进 JAK－STAT3 信号通路调控 SOCS3 的表达。

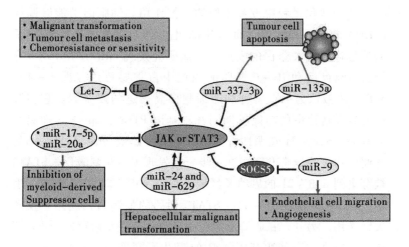

图 1－4 参与调控 JAK/STAT 通路的 miRNAs

（引自 Nat Rev Cancer, 2014, 14: 736－746）

综上所述，在炎症刺激下，IL－6 信号通路在多种肿瘤中通过不同的信号通路调控激活 STAT3，并维持其激活状态，进而促进肿瘤的恶性转化和恶性表型的维持。那么在胃癌中，Hp 感染造成的炎症诱发的 IL－6－STAT3 通路激活发挥如何的作用？其机制如何？

二、STAT3 是胃癌发生的关键信号通路

（一）IL-6 介导 Hp 感染导致胃癌的过程

多种研究表明，IL-6 是胃癌的重要驱动因素。流行病学研究表明，IL-6 同胃癌患者的预后相关。胃癌患者血清高水平的 IL-6 是一个独立的预后危险因素。IL-6 和 IL-11 在胃癌患者的胃黏膜中表达明显升高，而且同肿瘤的恶性表型密切相关，并影响预后。在胃癌的另一项研究中，IL-11 受体同肿瘤血管浸润和侵袭有关。STAT3 的激活同样同胃癌患者较差的预后相关。研究表明 STAT3 的激活，导致胃癌发生并促进胃癌细胞增殖的机制可能同 IL-11 的诱导有关。Hp 的感染是启动大部分胃癌的主要原因，而 Hp 的主要致病毒力蛋白 CagA 能够同 SHP-2 结合，引发异常的 ERK（胞外信号调节激酶）信号通路激活。胃黏膜感染 Hp 后，尤其是 CagA 阳性的 Hp，能够发生持续的 ERK 信号通路的激活，但同样激活了 STAT3 的和 IL-11 的产生。

动物实验也证实了 IL-6 在胃癌发生、发展中的重要作用。研究者构建了 Gp130 的转基因小鼠，发现在 3 个月后胃黏膜出现了异型增生和腺瘤。这类小鼠中由于缺乏 SOCS3 的抑制作用，因而出现了 STAT3 和 STAT1 的异常激活。Gp130 的配体 IL-6 和 IL-11 在这些小鼠的肿瘤中表达明显增加。而且，胃癌中 STAT3 和 Smad3 以及 mTORC1 等通路也存在上下游关系。另外，在多种小鼠胃癌模型中的研究发现，IL-11 的 mRNA 在肿瘤组织中明显升高；而对小鼠给予 IL-11 的缓慢刺激也能够在贲门

和胃窦部位诱发癌前病变；胃癌患者的肿瘤组织中 IL－11 表达明显升高。这些结果表明 IL－11 在胃癌发生中的重要作用。近期研究发现，IL－6 在人和小鼠胃癌组织中的间质纤维细胞中广泛存在，而且胃癌的致癌物 N－甲基－N－亚硝基脲在 IL－6 敲除的小鼠中不能诱发肿瘤。这些研究强烈提示 IL－6 和 IL－11 在胃黏膜上皮恶性转化和胃癌恶性表型进展中发挥了关键作用。

（二） STAT3 持续激活是胃癌发生的驱动因素

1. STAT3 激活诱发胃癌

胃癌的小鼠模型可以分为炎症型和非炎症型。炎症型胃癌模型一般而言是由 Hp 感染引起的，具有其他的基因型改变的背景，包括胃泌素高表达或者抑癌基因的缺失。其他的模型有肺 Hp 感染造成的基因组改变和慢性炎症，如 gp130^{7575FF} 突变，Ⅱ类 MHC（主要组织相溶性复合体）突变，IL－1β 过表达，以及 COX－2－2/PGES1 过表达。

在其中，gp130 突变小鼠的胃癌模型的将研究者兴趣引入到 STAT3 激活在胃癌中的意义。这种转基因鼠是在 gp130 的 757 酪氨酸位点进行突变后敲入小鼠，而 gp130 是 IL－6 家族的共受体。这样的突变阻止了配体结合后下游的 SHP－2 和 SOCS3 募集，进而导致 RAS/ERK/AP－1 信号通路的抑制。SOCS3 通常发挥负反馈抑制 STAT3 的功能，而当上述突变造成 SOCS3 的负反馈功能消失后，STAT3 就会出现持续的异常激活。因此，小鼠胃远端迅速出现了组织学同人胃癌进展阶段非常类似的肿瘤。这些阶段特征同 Correa 胃癌发生模式类似，包括胃炎、萎缩、黏液肠化生、不典型增生和黏膜侵袭，但并未出现转移。在这个模型中，STAT3 的活性形式显著升高对肿瘤的进展极为重要。STAT3 的基因敲除小鼠会导致胚胎死亡，但 gp130 突变同时有

STAT3 单倍体敲除的小鼠形成的胃癌肿瘤大小明显减低。

在 gp130 突变小鼠中，如果 gp130 不被激活，STAT3 的激活和肿瘤发生也不会出现。IL-11 也是 gp130 的配体，其在该模型中是不可或缺的刺激因素，这是因为如果在该小鼠模型中进一步敲除 IL-11 的共受体 IL-11 受体 α，则 STAT3 不会激活，肿瘤发生率也明显降低。对 gp130 突变小鼠采取无菌饲养和抗生素处理，结果发现 STAT3 的激活程度降低，肿瘤发生率也显著下降。因此，STAT3 的激活对于 gp130 突变小鼠胃癌发生至关重要，这依赖于 IL-11 同受体 gp130 的结合及胃的微生物环境。

在其他不依赖于 gp130 突变的胃癌模型中同样发现 STAT3 的异常激活和 IL-11 的表达。胃泌素缺乏的小鼠在 12 个月后能够发生胃癌，同时伴有萎缩、炎症和化生。这种肿瘤中能够检测出 IFN-γ 介导的炎症造成的 STAT3 激活。此外，缺少炎症刺激因素条件下，STAT3 激活和肿瘤发生的情况均明显减弱。有趣的是，在高胃泌素血症的小鼠中同样出现了 gp130 激活和下游的 STAT3 异常激活。敲除 H^+-K^+-ATP 酶后，小鼠出现胃酸缺乏，高胃泌素血症以及肿瘤形成，同时有 IL-11 表达升高和 STAT3 激活。此外，自身免疫性胃炎小鼠模型被发现有 IL-11 表达升高和 STAT3 激活。最后，过表达 COX-2、K19-C2mE 以及 K19-Wnt1C2mE 的转基因小鼠均能够出现胃底肿瘤，以及 IL-11 表达和 STAT3 激活。因此虽然启动胃癌发生的分子众多，但目前为止多数小鼠模型均能观察到 STAT3 激活引发的炎症反应。近期研究进一步支持了该观点，研究者通过小鼠尾静脉注射 IL-11 持续 7 天的方法发现胃黏膜出现炎症和胃底的明显萎缩。

2. STAT3 的激活机制

Hp 是胃癌发生的重要危险因素。许多研究证明宿主对 Hp 感染的反应是细菌、胃上皮细胞、免疫细胞三者之间通过一系列细胞因子及其受体和细胞内信号通路转导介导的。目前的观点多认为胃上皮细胞和浸润的免疫细胞均能够产生炎症因子，并维持慢性炎症状态，最终导致胃癌。众多信号通路中，STAT3 的激活是研究最为深入的之一，但 STAT3 活性对于 Hp 感染的免疫反应的作用及其是否介导了细菌引起的恶性转化等问题仍然不清楚。

STAT3 在胃黏膜和免疫系统中均发挥重要作用。通过控制细胞内特异的分子事件发生，STAT3 介导了黏膜慢性感染 Hp 过程中炎症变化和肿瘤发生机制。Hp 的 CagA 蛋白同 STAT3 的激活关系最为密切。

CagA 从 Hp 穿入胃上皮细胞后，定位于细胞膜内层，其 C 端的酪氨酸位点会被 src 和 c – Abl 激酶磷酸化。CagA 被证实在穿入细胞后同多条信号通路相互联系，这些通路多与细胞生长和运动有关（图 1 – 5）。目前认为 SHP – 2 是 CagA 最被广泛研究的细胞内靶分子。磷酸化的 CagA 能够特异性结合和激活 SHP2，导致 SHP – 2/RAS/ERK 信号通路的激活，进而异常调控细胞的极性和运动。另外，小干扰 RNA 沉默 SHP2 能够抑制 CagA 诱导的 ERK 活化。因此，SHP2 是 CagA 在胃上皮细胞中的关键介导分子。

SHP2 同 gp130 信号通路的联系使我们不能不考虑 STAT3 在 CagA 促进胃癌机制中的重要角色。研究者发现，CagA 阳性 Hp 感染的胃癌患者胃上皮中出现 STAT3 的显著激活。这为 STAT3 和 CagA 之间的联系提供了证据，并进一步为 CagA 在胃上皮细胞中驱动 STAT3 磷酸化提供了理论基础。近期研究发现，CagA 的磷酸化是 STAT3 激活的必要条件，这是由于将 CagA 的这些酪氨酸位点突变为丝氨酸后，CagA 诱导的 STAT3 激活现象被消除。另外两项研究同样证实了类似的结论。

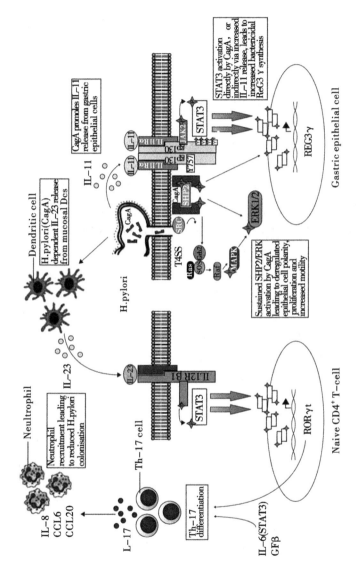

图1-5 CagA通过STAT3调控胃黏膜炎症的发生
（引自Expert Opin Ther Targets, 2012, 16: 889—901）

Hp 的另一个毒力因素 VacA 能够通过激活 Bcl – 2 家族蛋白而导致胃上皮细胞的凋亡。STAT3 的功能是抑制凋亡，因而 VacA 在胃癌细胞系中导致的 STAT3 抑制及 Bcl – 2 和 Bcl – XL 并不意外。虽然在体内 STAT3 同 VacA 的关系尚不明确，但是慢性 Hp 感染在人和小鼠模型中造成的 STAT3 激活表明 VacA 对 STAT3 的抑制作用可能被 Hp 的其他机制所掩盖。

3. STAT3 引发胃上皮细胞基因改变

STAT3 已知能够转录调控许多靶基因。研究者深入探索了胃癌中 gp130/STAT3 通路驱动的基因谱。目前普遍认为大部分胃癌的发生部位远端胃对 IL – 11 反应敏感，后者特异性激活 STAT 而不影响 MAPK/ERK 通路。IL – 11/STAT3 激活的基因谱可分为两类：胃窦和胃体部。胃窦部早期基因改变，包括 Reg 家族基因、Clusterin、Gremlin – 1、gp130、SOCS3、Jak1、Timp1 和 Gas1。

相比之下，胃体黏膜的基因改变则更为多样化，主要包括：①增殖相关基因，如 Reg 家族基因、Igfbp4、Gsdmc1、Grem1 和 Blm1；②免疫相关基因，如 SerpinA 家族基因、Dmbt1、IL – 33、Spp1、MyD88 等；③信号转导基因，如 Socs3、Jak3 和 Jun b。这些基因中大部分均被报道同肿瘤相关，尤其是 Reg 家族蛋白、Blm1 和 Grem1。

不少其他研究也在胃癌中间接探讨了 STAT3 的调控基因。研究发现，STAT3 的激活同 VEGF、c – Myc、Survivin、MMP – 7、CD44v6 和 CyclinD1 等相关，这些靶基因中大部分也相继在小鼠模型中被证实。其他研究还发现 survivin 和 Bcl – 2 的表达依赖于 STAT3 的激活。总而言之，胃黏膜上皮中一系列基因被 STAT3 直接调控，这些基因在胃上皮细胞恶性转化过程中起了推动作用。

三、CypB 同 STAT3 功能关系密切

（一）Cyclophillin 家族基因

亲环素蛋白（cyclophilins）是一组具有肽基脯氨酰异构酶活性的蛋白。这类蛋白能够将含有脯氨酸的肽链由顺式转化为反式，同时能够辅助蛋白折叠。该蛋白在原核和真核细胞中均广泛表达，最早在 1984 年被发现是环孢素 A 的细胞内结合蛋白。但是 5 年后的 1989 年才发现这个蛋白其实同 18 kDa 的、具有肽基脯氨酰异构酶活性的 CypA 事实上是同一种蛋白。

目前为止，一共有 17 种亲环素蛋白在人类基因组被发现，但其中大部分蛋白的功能尚不明确，只有 7 中亲环素蛋白具有异构酶活性或能够结合环孢素 A。亲环素家族蛋白具有一个含有 109 个氨基酸的共同结构域，即亲环素样结构域。这个核心结构域周围被特异性的结构域所围绕，这些结构域决定了不同类型亲环素家族蛋白在细胞内的定位和功能。一部分亲环素家族蛋白的定位已经被陆续鉴定，如 CypA 和 Cyp40 主要在细胞质溶胶中，CypB 和 CypC 位于内质网的膜上，CypD 位于线粒体，CypE 和 CypA 在细胞核内被发现，CypNK 主要在 NK 细胞中出现。

在过去 20 年中，许多研究重点被放在 CypA、CypB 和 CypD 上，这是由于这些蛋白同特异性的细胞功能和疾病进展有密切关系；而其他亲环素家族蛋白的特点和在疾病进展中发挥的作用则尚不明确。CypA 是细胞质中丰度最高的蛋白之一，其含量约占细胞质总蛋白含量的 0.1%，其功能同细胞内蛋白的折叠、

运输、免疫修饰和细胞信号转导有关。CypA 在炎症刺激或 ROS 反应下能够被自发的从细胞分泌，而细胞外的 CypA 碎片能够作为炎症介导因子促进炎症反应并通过细胞表面受体 CD147 发挥对中性粒细胞和单核细胞的调控作用。一些研究发现，CypA 的基因敲除小鼠和沉默的细胞系相关的实验表明 CypA 在细胞增殖和存活中意义并不大。CypA 的表达上升在多种病理过程中发挥作用，如肺纤维化过程中炎症反应、类风湿关节炎中的炎症反应和软骨破坏、ROS 和炎症的恶化。近期研究也发现 CypA 在肿瘤细胞中表达升高并促进转移。

CypD 是另一个关键亲环素家族蛋白，其定位于线粒体，能够调控线粒体通透性转换孔（mitochondrial permeability transition pore，MPTP）。因此它被认为在线粒体功能失常导致的多种疾病中具有作为药物靶点的潜能。线粒体被认为是控制细胞不同部位钙离子浓度的防火墙。线粒体外膜上的钙离子主要通过电压依赖的离子通道（voltage–dependent anion channel，VDAC）运输。当 MPTP 开放时，钙离子迅速从线粒体向细胞质外流，产生钙离子信号。一些肝细胞、神经元或心肌细胞的研究证实 CypD 是 MPTP 开放的关键调控因子。持续的 MPTP 的开放导致细胞出现不同于细胞坏死性凋亡的一种坏死状死亡，这种死亡由 RIPK3 介导。近期发现线粒体通透性增加造成的细胞坏死通过两种不同的信号通路介导，而两种途径的同时抑制——如 CypD 的抑制和 RIPK1 抑制——能够对缺血再灌注损伤进行保护。

（二）CypB 的功能

CypB 是第二个被鉴定的亲环素蛋白。它同 CypA 的不同点在于其 N 端具有一个可切除序列，用于引导蛋白进入内质网。环孢素 A 和其他亲环素抑制剂能够特异性改变 CypB 的亚细胞定位，将其从内质网移除，并促进它向细胞外的分泌。同CypB不同，CypA在抑制剂作用下不会分泌到细胞外。细胞外的CypA和CypB碎片同细胞间信号转导和炎症反应有关，但单独的CypB似乎不能诱导炎症相关细胞因子的产生。CypB在病毒感染等疾病中发挥宿主的介导作用。

1. CypB是调控丙型肝炎的病毒RNA聚合酶的调控分子

病毒复制依赖宿主的基因组来源的相关分子的调控。研究者发现细胞内的CypB对于HCV（丙型肝炎病毒）基因组复制的复制效率至关重要。CypB同HCV的RNA聚合酶NS5B结合并直接促进它同RNA结合活性。通过小干扰RNA沉默内源性CypB表达的方式能够降低HCV复制的效率，而且通过其他方式诱导NS5B结合CypB也得到了同样的结果。因此CypB是HCV复制相关复合体的关键调控因子，这项研究为CypB作为抗病毒治疗的靶点提供了理论基础。

2. CypB细胞内的催乳素/CypB复合体促进转录

催乳素的细胞核内转运机制被广泛研究。催乳素被认为同CypB结合，后者介导了催乳素的促进增殖、细胞生长和细胞核内的催乳速运输等过程。将CypB的PPI（肽基脯氨酰基顺反异构酶）活性结构域移除后，这些现象则消失。研究者发现，细胞核内的催乳素/CypB复合体能够直接同STAT5结合，导致STAT抑制剂PIAS3的表达降低，进而促进STAT5同DNA结合发挥对下游靶基因的转录调控作用。

（三）CypB与肿瘤

CypB被发现在多种肿瘤中发挥促癌作用。

1. CypB与胰腺癌

研究者收集了肿瘤细胞培养液的上清液并分析其中的蛋白

组分，发现 **CypB** 在其中明显升高。随后将 **CypB** 作为血清标志物，检验胰腺癌患者血清中 CypB 的含量，结果证实这种检测方法具有作为胰腺癌诊断的潜力。

2. CypB 和乳腺癌

研究者在乳腺癌细胞中通过 RNAi 技术沉默了 CypB 的表达，随后发现 663 个转录本被 CypB 调控，而这些基因中大部分同细胞增殖、运动和肿瘤恶性表型相关。进一步通过 PCR 验证发现 STMN3、S100A4、S100A6、c - Myb 等基因都随 CypB 的沉默而表达下降。接下来的功能实验证实 CypB 的下调降低了细胞增殖、生长和运动。细胞免疫荧光和免疫组织化学实验发现在配对的乳腺癌组织中，CypB 的表达同乳腺癌的进展密切相关。这些结果提示 CypB 在乳腺癌中可能通过调控细胞增殖和运动促进恶性表型进展。另一项乳腺癌的研究也发现，CypB 参与调控催乳素引起的乳腺癌的发生和发展。其机制可能同乳腺癌相关的基因表达、癌细胞生长增殖和运动有关。

3. CypB 与骨髓瘤

研究者在骨髓瘤中发现，CypB 同 STAT3 功能相关，而同家族的成员 CypA 则不明显。CypB 的沉默抑制了 IL - 6 诱导的 STAT3 转录活性，而不影响 STAT3 的磷酸化。CypB 被发现能够结合 STAT3 的靶分子启动子区，而且沉默 CypB 后 STAT3 的细胞内定位出现了变化，这说明 CypB 同 STAT3 在细胞核内的功能有密切关系。相比之下，CypA 的沉默抑制了 IL - 6 诱导的 STAT3 磷酸化和细胞核内转位。Cyp 的抑制剂环孢素 A 的使用造成了类似的结果。但是 IL - 6 造成的 STAT1 的激活并不会被 Cyp 的沉默所影响。结果，Cyp 的沉默造成了 IL - 6 通路向 STAT1 下游信号通路倾斜。此外，Cyp 的删除或环孢素 A 的使用促进了 IL - 6 依赖的多发骨髓瘤细胞的凋亡，但 IL - 6 不依赖的细胞系则不受影响。因此 Cyp 蛋白促进了 STAT3 的抑制凋亡作用。总而言之，CypB 和 CypA 在肿瘤中通过不同方面发挥重要功能。

4．CypB 与头颈肿瘤

研究者发现在头颈部肿瘤中 CypB 的表达同放疗的敏感性相关。通过小干扰 RNA 沉默 CypB 或者环孢素 A 抑制 CypB 后发现肿瘤细胞的放疗敏感性明显升高，而 DNA 损伤修复降低。通过免疫组化对 CypB 在患者肿瘤组织中的水平可见 CypB 的表达同放疗后的疗效有明显相关关系。

5．CypB 与肝癌

研究者在肝癌中研究了缺氧环境诱导 CypB 表达的功能和机制。结果发现，HIF-1α 在缺氧环境下诱导 CypB 的产生。有趣的是，CypB 能够保护肿瘤细胞抵抗缺氧和顺铂诱导的细胞凋亡。进一步研究发现，CypB 在血管生成和葡萄糖代谢等过程中能够反馈性调控 HIF-1α 的表达。研究者还在体内实验中验证了 CypB 调控肿瘤化疗耐药的功能。最后，肿瘤组织中研究 CypB 的表达结果证实 CypB 在78%的肝癌和91%的结肠癌组织中均表达明显升高，且其表达同肿瘤患者的预后相关。另一项研究发现 CypB 在肝癌细胞中能够同受体 CD147 结合，从而保护细胞抵抗氧化应激反应。

6．CypB 与胶质瘤

研究者发现 CypB 向胶质瘤细胞提供关键的存活相关信号通路。功能实验发现 CypB 的低表达在体内和体外抑制细胞增殖和存活，随后发现 CypB 抑制剂环孢素 A 的使用得到同样的结果。抑制 CypB 的表达引起 Ras 信号通路的过度激活、细胞衰老信号的诱导，以及 MYC、突变型 P53、JAK/STAT3 信号通路的丢失。在 CypB 沉默的胶质瘤细胞中可观察到 ROS 增加、内质网扩展以及异常的未折叠的蛋白增多，这表明 CypB 抑制 ROS 和内质网应激。CypB 下游的促进细胞存活的突变癌基因表达可能是胶质瘤预后较差的原因。

由此可见，CypB 在多种肿瘤中高表达，且同 STAT3 的激活和下游基因的转录功能密切相关。那么胃癌中 CypB 的表达如何？其功能是否同 STAT3 在 Hp 感染和炎症反应刺激条件下持续的激活有关？这些问题将是我们研究的重点。

（四）　CypB 受调控机制

从以上研究不难看出，CypB 在肿瘤中表达异常增高。那么 CypB 的上游受到何种信号通路调控？一些研究就这个问题进行了探讨。

1. CypB 与转录因子

研究者发现，CypB 的表达受到缺氧条件的诱导。首先，HIF-1α 能够在缺氧条件下直接促进 CypB 的转录。研究发现肝癌细胞在缺氧环境培养 12 小时后，CypB 的 mRNA 和蛋白水平均表达增高，且增高趋势有时间依赖性。而对肝癌细胞系采用 HIF-1α 诱导剂 $COCl_2$ 或 DFO 刺激后 CypB 的表达同样增高明显。双荧光素酶报告基因实验证实，HIF-1α 在缺氧条件下被诱导表达之后能够直接结合 CypB 的启动子区，促进后者的转录。这些实验表明 HIF-1α 能够促进 CypB 的转录和表达。

2. CypB 与转录后修饰

CHOP（CCAAT/enhancer-binding protein-homologous protein，CCAAT/增强子结合蛋白同源蛋白）是内质网应激的效应因子，其在肿瘤细胞存活中发挥重要作用。缺氧环境是通过内质网导致细胞死亡的重要应激刺激，尤其在实体肿瘤中。研究者发现在缺氧条件下，CypB 同 P300 结合能够促进 CHOP 的泛素化和蛋白更新。研究发现 CypB 能够直接结合 CHOP 的 N 端 α 螺旋结构域并同 P300 配合诱导 CHOP 的泛素化。研究者还发现在缺氧条件下 CypB 被 ATF6 促进转录。因此，CypB 通过调控 CHOP 的泛素化修饰影响 CHOP 降解，进而抑制了缺氧造成的细胞死亡。

3. MicroRNA

MicroRNA 是近年来研究逐渐深入的具有重要调控功能的小分子。其通过碱基互补序列识别或者结合靶基因 miRNA 的非编码区域，发挥抑制靶基因编码蛋白表达的表观调控作用。MicroRNA 最早被发现在低等生物的分化和发育过程中发挥重要作用。在肿瘤中，miRNA 通过对靶基因的调控影响多种肿瘤的恶性表型。而胃癌中 CypB 的异常表达同 miRNA 的关系尚无研究探讨。

（五）MicroRNA-520d-5p 可能参与调控 CypB

1. MicroRNA 是调控胃癌增殖的关键因素

许多研究发现，miRNA 被发现在癌症包括胃癌的发生和发展中也发挥了不可忽视的作用。首先，大多数肿瘤组织中 miRNA 的表达同癌旁正常组织相比具有显著的差异。针对 B 细胞淋巴瘤的研究发现，13 号染色体位点扩增导致 miR-17-92 簇表达显著增加，胃癌、肝癌、乳腺癌等恶性肿瘤中 miRNA 的表达谱出现了紊乱，提示 miRNA 表达失调可能与肿瘤的发生、发展密切相关；目前已知的 miRNA 一半以上位于肿瘤相关基因位点，如染色体断裂位点、杂合性缺失和脆性位点（fragile sites）等等，提示 miRNA 表达紊乱是肿瘤发生的关键分子变化；此外，联合 7 个 microRNA 可以较好预测胃癌患者的生存率和复发率，这说明表达异常的 microRNA 可能影响肿瘤患者的预后；最重要的是，人为调控 microRNA 在肿瘤组织中的表达，可以有效抑制肿瘤恶性表型。在胶质瘤中上调 miR-128 能显著抑制增殖和自我更新。这些证据共同表明，microRNA 同肿瘤包括胃癌的发生、发展密切相关，且具有良好的应用价值。

那么 CypB 在胃癌中表达异常变化是否同 miRNA 的表达失调有关呢？MicroRNA 是否在 Hp 感染造成的炎症引发胃癌的病理过程中参与了 CypB 的调控呢？

2. miR - 520d - 5p 是抑癌基因

通过生物信息学研究方法，我们发现 miR - 520d - 5p 是潜在的 CypB 的调控 miRNA。既往研究表示，miR - 520d - 5p 是一个抑癌 miRNA。

研究发现，在乳腺癌中 miR - 520 家族 miRNA 可能通过直接靶向 RELA 强烈抑制 NF - κB 通路，并降低炎症因子 IL - 6 和 IL - 8 的表达和分泌。通过体内和体外实验，研究者发现 miR - 520 家族基因能够抑制乳腺癌细胞转移，基因芯片的结果表明这些 miRNA 发挥功能的机制可能同 TGF - β 信号通路有关。进一步研究发现，miR - 520/373 的抑制转移功能由其对靶分子 TGF - β 受体的直接抑制介导。miR - 520 同 TGFBR2 的表达在 ER 阴性的乳腺癌患者组织中负相关，而在 ER 阳性的患者中则无相关。值得注意的是，miR - 520 表达降低同 ER 阴性的肿瘤淋巴结转移有关。这些结果表明 miR - 520 家族基因在乳腺癌中发挥抑制炎症信号通路和转移的作用。

另一项研究发现，miR - 520 在肝癌中也是一个抑癌基因。代谢变化在多种肿瘤中均被发现且同患者的临床转归有关。因此肿瘤细胞中的代谢异常信号通路可能是肿瘤治疗的靶点。研究表明，肝癌中 TARDBP（Tat - activating regulatory DNA - binding protein，达激活调节性 DNA 结合蛋白）调控 PFK（phosphofructokinase，磷酸果糖激酶）的表达，后者是糖酵解和葡萄糖分解过程中的限速酶。抑制 TARDBP 的表达后，肝癌细胞会出现葡萄糖的分解受阻，进而生长受抑。有趣的是，miR - 520 家族基因是 TARDBP 介导的糖酵解过程中的中间调节因子。TARDBP能够抑制 miR-520 的表达，而后者抑制 PFK 的表达。研究最终在肝癌组织中验证了 TARDBP 同肝癌患者预后的关系。这些结果表明 miR-520 在肝癌中能够通过调控肿瘤代谢抑制肿瘤增殖。

另一项在肝癌中的研究指出，miR-520d 能够增加肝癌细胞对 5-氟尿嘧啶（5-FU）的敏感性。研究发现，EGFR 突变体Ⅲ能够促抑制 miR-520d 的表达，进而导致转录因子 E2F-1 和胸腺嘧啶合成酶 TS 的表达升高，后二者是介导肝癌耐药的重要调控因素。研究者发现 EGFRVⅢ的抗体 CH12 和 5-FU 联合使用能够对肝癌有加成的治疗作用，并延长了荷瘤小鼠的生存时间。有趣的是，CH12的使用能够增加 miR-520d 的表达，并进而导致 E2F-1 和 TS 的mRNA 及蛋白的水平降低。这些结果表明，miR-520d 在肝癌中具有作为增加化疗敏感性的潜在治疗价值。

近期研究发现，miR-520d-5p 能够通过靶向 TWIST1 抑制肿瘤转移。研究表明 miR-520d-5p 靶向 TWIST1 的 UTR 区域，进一步研究发现 miR-520d-5p 导致的 TWIST1 表达抑制能够造成后者下游的 miR-10b 的表达降低，进而能够 E-钙黏素（E-cadherin）的表达升高，从而抑制肿瘤细胞发生 EMT，抑制肿瘤转移。此外，研究者还发现 miR-520d-5p 还能够抑制肿瘤细胞的增殖，而且高水平的 miR-520d-5p 同肿瘤患者的生存期延长有关。这些结果表明 miR-520d-5p 能够抑制肿瘤的增殖和转移，是抑癌基因。

miR-520d-5p 还被发现在结肠癌中调控肿瘤的转移和增殖。研究通过 qRT-PCR 证实，同癌旁正常组织相比，miR-520d-5p在结肠癌组织中表达明显降低。双荧光素酶报告基因研究表明，miR-520d-5p 能够靶向 CTHRC1（collagen triple helix repeat containing 1），并受到 SP1 的直接转录促进调控。在结肠癌主细胞中过表达 miR – 520d – 5p 能够抑制肿瘤增殖、转移和侵袭。而 miR – 520d – 5p 的沉默则在体内和体外实验中均得到相反的结果。WB 结果表明，miR – 520d – 5p 通过抑制 ERK1/2 激活而抑制 EMT 的发生。可见，在结肠癌中 miR – 520d – 5p 能够通过抑制肿瘤增殖和转移等恶性表型发挥抑癌作用。

3. miR – 520d – 5p 可能在胃癌中参与调控 CypB

我们通过生物信息学预测，发现 miR – 520d – 5p 可能在 CypB 的 3′ – UTR 具有潜在结合靶点。而在组织和细胞中验证 miR – 520d – 5p 同 CypB 的表达，结果表明二者的表达在胃癌组织和细胞中呈负相关关系。这些结果强烈提示 miR – 520d – 5p 可能是 CypB 在胃癌中表达异常的原因之一。

因此，本研究聚焦 CypB 在胃癌中的功能及其上下游信号通路，旨在进一步理解 Hp 感染和炎症刺激引发胃癌的机制，为胃癌的诊治新策略提供思路。

四、CypB/STAT3/miR – 520d – 5p 反馈环路促进胃癌增殖

前期研究发现 CypB 的表达上调可能促进了乳腺癌、骨髓瘤、肝癌以及胶质瘤的恶性进展，这主要是由于 CypB 促进细胞通过产生 ROS 以存活以及 STAT3 的核转位及下游分子的表达。而 CypB 在胃癌发生、发展过程中的表达和功能迄今为止尚无明确定论。在本部分研究中，我们发现胃癌中 CypB 的表达显著上调，且沉默 CypB 后，胃癌细胞的体内和体外生长均受到抑制，这与既往的其他肿瘤中的研究所得结论基本一致。

（一）CypB 在胃癌表达升高且促进胃癌生长

CypB 在肿瘤中的研究最早由 Fang 等在乳腺癌中进行。研究者通过转染 siRNA 对 CypB 进行沉默后进行了表达谱芯片的分析发现 663 个基因在 CypB 沉默后发生明显表达变化，而其中许多基因都同细胞的生长增殖、运动能力等有密切关系，功能实验也证实了 CypB 沉默后细胞的生长、运动均显著降低。随后一项肝癌中的研究指出，肝癌的缺氧环境导致的 HIF-1α 激活能够诱导 CypB 的产生，后者对于缺氧和顺铂诱导的细胞凋亡具有显著的保护作用。此外骨髓瘤和胶质瘤中的研究结果也证实 CypB对于维持肿瘤细胞增殖、抑制细胞凋亡具有重要作用。这些研究都认为 CypB 的表达异常升高是相应肿瘤的特性，而且功能实验也证实抑制 CypB 在相应肿瘤中的表达能够抑制细胞生长，造成细胞凋亡。因而抑制 CypB 表达可能是一种重要的抑制肿瘤进展的策略。

胃癌是我国发病率、死亡率排名前列的肿瘤，而目前为止尚无研究阐明 CypB 在胃癌中的表达和功能。在本部分研究中，我们首先通过免疫组化实验证实胃癌组织中 CypB 的表达升高，还发现高水平 CypB 的患者生存期缩短，该表型是胃癌患者预后较差的危险因素。此外，作为分泌蛋白，CypB 能够在血清中被检出。我们因此同时探索了胃癌患者血清中 CypB 浓度的诊断价值。结果发现同正常人血清中 CypB 浓度相比，胃癌患者血清中的 CypB 的浓度显著升高；更有意思的是，将受检的胃癌患者按照 TNM 分期进行分组发现，T_3 和 T_4 期胃癌的患者具有相对较高的血清 CypB 浓度，且发生淋巴结转移的胃癌患者血清 CypB 的浓度也相对较高。近期另一项胰腺癌的研究也发现，胰腺癌患者血清中 CypB 浓度也显著高于志愿者。这项研究设计的适配子能够特异性结合多种胰腺癌细胞系的培养液上清，研究者进一步通过蛋白质谱技术检测发现其适配子结合的正是 CypB。综合我们的结果可知，同既往研究结论类似，CypB 在胃癌中表达升高，且高水平表达的 CypB 是独立的预后危险因素；此外，CypB 具有对胃癌的血清学诊断具有重要潜在价值。

为了进一步探索胃癌中 CypB 的功能，我们首先检测了几株胃癌细胞系及正常胃上皮细胞系中 CypB 的表达，发现胃癌细胞中 CypB 的表达明显升高，这也支持了之前在胃癌组织中进行的免疫组织化学实验结果。我们挑选了 CypB 表达相对较高的 SGC7901 和 BGC823 细胞进行功能缺失模型建立，随后进行的体内外功能实验均发现 CypB 沉默后，胃癌细胞的生长明显减缓。抑制 CypB 表达，胃癌细胞发生 G_0/G_1 期的细胞周期阻滞，且凋亡率明显升高。这些结果证明 CypB 的异常表达可能是胃癌维持增殖，克服凋亡的重要基础。那么，胃癌中 CypB 的表达通过何种机制促进胃癌的增殖和存活呢？我们在下一部分中着重讨论了这个问题。

（二）CypB 通过激活 STAT3 促进胃癌增殖

在上一部分中，我们发现 CypB 的表达在胃癌组织和细胞中以及胃癌患者的血清中异常增高，而且沉默 CypB 的表达能够在体内外抑制胃癌细胞的增殖，促进胃癌细胞的凋亡。那么 CypB 调控胃癌增殖的机制如何？

近期几项研究分别从不同方面阐述了 CypB 在肿瘤中的功能，证明 CypB 在骨髓瘤、肝癌、胶质瘤、乳腺癌等肿瘤中促进肿瘤增殖、抑制凋亡。而近期研究则发现肿瘤细胞中 CypB 的表达是 STAT3 激活的必要条件。在骨髓瘤中，CypB 与激活的 STAT3 共定位，且 CypB 能促进 STAT3 的磷酸化；在恶性胶质瘤中，药物抑制 CypB 后 STAT3 的磷酸化受到抑。这些结果提示 CypB 在肿瘤中调控恶性表型的功能同 STAT3 的活化可能有密切关系。

那么，胃癌中 CypB 和 STAT3 的关系如何呢? 是否 CypB 调控胃癌增殖的功能是通过 STAT3 介导的呢? 带着这些问题，我们进行了第二部分研究。

本部分研究探讨了 CypB 和 STAT3 的激活在调控胃癌增殖过程中的相互关系。我们发现 CypB 和 pSTAT3 在胃癌组织中均表达上调，且二者的表达呈正相关关系。随后我们进一步在胃癌细胞系中证实: 过表达 CypB 后，STAT3 的磷酸化增多; 相反，沉默 CypB 后，STAT3 的磷酸化水平则降低。这些结果提示 CypB 可能在胃癌组织中的 STAT3 激活过程中具有重要作用。此外我们还发现一个有趣的现象: 作为 STAT3 信号通路的经典启动因子，IL-6 的刺激能够引发 STAT3 的磷酸化和入核，但与此同时正常情况下大部分定位于内质网的 CypB 也伴随 STAT3 进入了细胞核。这些结果强烈提示 CypB 对于 STAT3 在包括磷酸化和进入细胞核在内的活化过程中可能具有重要功能。

近期几项研究也支持该结论。Bauer 等发现在骨髓瘤中 CypB 能特异性同 STAT3 结合，他们使用 siRNA 对 CypB 进行干扰沉默后发现 IL-6 刺激引起的 STAT3 的核转位受到了明显抑制，CypB 的特异性抑制剂环孢霉素 A 的使用也产生了类似的结果; 此外 CypB 被发现同 STAT3 的靶分子的启动子区能够结合，这表明 CypB 在伴随 STAT3 进入细胞核后进一步发挥转录功能有密切关系。Choi 等在胶质瘤中同样发现，抑制 CypB 后，细胞会发生 RAS/MAPK 通路的过度激活，以及细胞衰老信号通路的激活; 细胞的 CypB 表达抑制后还发生大量凋亡，其原因包括 MYC、突变型 P53、Chk1 以及 JAK/STAT3 信号通路的受阻。综合这些结果可见，在骨髓瘤和胶质瘤中 CypB 是一个促癌基因，其功能可能通过 STAT3 信号通路激活发挥；而我们的实验数据在胃癌中也证实了 STAT3 磷酸化、入核及发挥促进转录的功能均需要 CypB 的辅助。

为研究 STAT3 的激活是否在胃癌中介导了 CypB 功能的发挥，我们进一步采用了 STAT3 的 shRNA 进行研究。结果发现 CypB 的过表达促进胃癌生长，而沉默 STAT3 后，细胞增殖的促进作用被逆转，这证明 STAT3 可能是介导 CypB 发挥促进胃癌功能的下游分子。

结合我们的研究结果，可见 CypB 的表达异常增高，可能支持了 STAT3 的进一步激活，从而促进炎症反应慢性刺激过程中胃癌的发生。那么，CypB 的表达升高原因是什么？

（三）miR – 520d – 5p 通过靶向 CypB 调控胃癌增殖

在前两个部分中，我们发现 CypB 在胃癌组织和细胞中表达升高，且其促进胃癌增殖的功能发挥可能通过 STAT3 介导。但是 CypB 在胃癌组织中异常过表达的原因是什么？近期研究发现，研究者发现，CypB 的表达受到缺氧条件的诱导。HIF – 1α 能够在缺氧条件下直接促进 CypB 的转录。研究发现肝癌细胞在缺氧环境培养 12 小时后，CypB 的 mRNA 和蛋白水平均表达增高，且增高趋势有时间依赖性。此外，缺氧环境下 CypB 被 ATF6 促进转录。前者进而通过调控 CHOP 的泛素化修饰影响 CHOP 降解，进而抑制了缺氧造成的细胞死亡。

而 CypB 是否受到 microRNA 的调控，尚无文献报道。近期结果表明 miRNA 在胃癌的发生、发展中起了关键作用。因此我们在本部分中重点研究了可能参与调控 CypB 的 microRNA 及其在胃癌细胞中的功能。

我们通过体内和体外实验证实，CypB 是 miR – 520d – 5p 的靶基因，介导了后者在胃癌增殖和存活中的功能。

CypB 的表达调控目前研究较少，近期研究发现 miRNA 是一类重要表观遗传学调控分子，通过靶向靶基因 3'-UTR 抑制其表达。近期许多证据表明，microRNA 同肿瘤包括胃癌的发生、发展密切相关。那么 CypB 在胃癌中表达异常变化是否同 miRNA 的表达失调有关呢？MicroRNA 是否在 Hp 感染造成的炎症引发胃癌的病理过程中参与了 CypB 的调控呢？

我们通过生物信息预测发现 miR-520d-5p 是潜在的 CypB 上游调控 miRNA。细胞中二者表达负相关，提示 miR-520d-5p 的表达异常可能是 CypB 的表达失调的原因。近期多种研究也表明 miR-520d-5p 是抑癌 miRNA。

前文也述及 miR-520d-p 家族成员在多种肿瘤中发挥抑癌作用。结合我们的研究结果，我们可知在胃癌中 miR-520d-5p 同样是发挥抑癌作用。我们首先通过生物信息学分析我们筛选到若干可能调控 CypB 的 microRNA，并将其 mimics 分别转染胃癌细胞系。结果发现，miR-520d-5p 能够抑制 CypB 的表达。双荧光素酶报告基因实验证实，miR-520d-5p 能够直接结合 CypB 的 3'端非翻译区。QRT-PCR 和 Western Blotting 实验进一步证实，miR-520d-5p 在转录水平导致 CypB 的 miRNA 降解。这些实验证实，miR-520d-5p 是 CypB 上游的直接调控分子。这是首次从 miRNA 角度分析 CypB 的表达异常的研究，对于解释 CypB 在胃癌中表达异常变化具有重要意义。

随后我们研究了 miR-520d-5p 同其靶基因 CypB 在调控胃癌增殖过程中的功能。我们建立了 miR-520d-5p 的功能获得、缺失模型。随后的功能实验证实，无论在体内还是体外，miR-520d-5p 均抑制胃癌细胞增殖，促进细胞凋亡。随后含有野生型和突变性 3'-UTR 的 CypB 表达载体同 miR-520d-5p 被用于共感染细胞，XTT 和克隆形成实验表明 miR-520d-5p 能够减弱野生型 3′–UTR 的 CypB 载体对胃癌细胞增殖的促进作用，但不能逆转突变型 3′–UTR 的 CypB 载体的作用。流式细胞周期和凋亡分析实验得到了类似的结果。这进一步说明，miR–520d–5p 通过结合 CypB 3′–UTR 调控胃癌细胞生长。

总结本部分结果，我们探索了 miR–520d–5p/CypB 通路在胃癌中的功能，那么它们在胃癌炎癌转化中同 STAT3 激活的相关机制如何？

（四）miR–520d–5p 通过 CypB 调控 STAT3 活性

综合前面的结果，我们可以推断 CyPB 是 miR–520d–5p 的功能性靶基因，而 CypB 的功能发挥通过 STAT3 介导，那么是否 miR–520d–5p/CypB 轴能够在胃癌细胞中调控 STAT3 的活性呢？

在本部分研究中，我们进一步探索了 miR–520d–5p/CyPB 通路的下游机制。我们发现，miR–520d–5p 过表达抑制了 JAK2 和 STAT3 的磷酸化，而且 IL–6 刺激造成的 STAT3 磷酸化随时间和浓度的依赖性受到 miR–520d–5p 过表达的抑制。另外，IL–6 刺激能搞导致 CypB 和 STAT3 在细胞核的共定位；而 miR–520d–5p 介导 CypB 沉默后，STAT3 的入核受到了明显的抑制。随后的功能实验证实，STAT3 的敲除能够逆转 miR–520d–5p 的沉默对细胞生长和细胞周期、凋亡的影响。这些结果说明 miR–520d–5p 通过调控 CypB/STAT3 轴影响 STAT3 的活化和胃癌细胞增殖。我们的研究补充了 IL–6/STAT3 信号通路中 STAT3 的调控机制。证实 miR–520d–5p/STAT3 通路调控 STAT3 的激活，进而调控胃癌恶性表型。

（五）STAT3 直接抑制 miR-520d-5p 表达

作为转录因子，STAT3 能够直接促进或者抑制 miRNA 的表达，而 miRNA 反过来可能直接或者间接以 STAT3 信号通路相关蛋白为靶基因。

我们的研究发现，STAT3 直接抑制 miR-520d-5p 在胃癌细胞中的表达。为了进一步阐明 CypB 同 STAT3 活化之间的关系，我们对 GES-1 细胞采用 IL-6 的刺激，发现 STAT3 的磷酸化上调的同时，CypB 的表达也明显升高；而 miR-520d-5p 的过表达则能够抑制该现象发生，这提示 STAT3 可能反馈性参与 miR-520d-5p 的表达调控。QRT-PCR 结果证实，IL-6 刺激能够在胃癌细胞中造成 miR-520d-5p 表达的下调，而 STAT3 的 shRNA 则逆转该现象发生。随后生物信息学预测发现，miR-520d-5p 的启动子区域存在多个潜在的 STAT3 的结合位点。因此针对 STAT3 在不同位置的结合位点，我们建立了一系列 miR-520d-5p 启动子的截短载体。双荧光素酶报告基因实验证实 STAT3 的结合位点位于 -1329 至 -722bp。对该区域的两个结合位点分别或同时突变发现，当 -733 至 -723bp 区域发生突变时，STAT3 依赖的 miR-520d-5p 的调控出现缺失。染色质免疫共沉淀也证实 STAT3 蛋白能够同该区域 DNA 直接结合，而且经 IL-6 刺激后其结合的 DNA 增多。这些结果说明，STAT3 通过直接结合 miR-520d 的启动子区域，转录性抑制其表达。

因此，我们发现胃癌细胞中存在一条由 IL-6 炎症因子诱发的 CypB/STAT3/miR-520d-5p 正反馈通路。在癌症发生的过程中，转录因子同 miRNA 经常形成反馈通路，因为转录因子能够直接促进或抑制 miRNA 的表达，而前者同时有可能是后者的直接或者间接靶基因。这些反馈通路的形成,为胃上皮细胞在炎症刺激下的恶性转化提供了基础,并为肿瘤细胞维持恶性表型提供了先决条件。那么这条正反馈通路是否能够在胃癌组织中得到验证呢?

(六) 胃癌组织中存在 CypB/STAT3/miR – 520d – 5p

在本部分研究中,我们在胃癌组织中验证了 CypB/STAT3/miR – 520d – 5p 的反馈环路的表达。我们首先通过原位杂交结果发现,胃癌组织中 miR – 520d – 5p 的表达同癌旁组织相比明显降低,且低水平的 miR – 520d – 5p 患者预后较差,COX 多因素分析结果也显示低水平的 miR – 520d – 5p 是独立预后因素。此外,我们将 90 例胃癌患者按照 miR – 520d – 5p、CypB 及 pSTAT3 的表达水平高低进行分组和相关分析,发现低水平的 miR – 520d – 5p 同 CypB 及 pSTAT3 的表达升高有相关关系。因此,我们在组织中验证了 CypB/STAT3/miR – 520d – 5p 反馈环路的存在,证明了 IL – 6/STAT3 信号通路通过影响 miR – 520d – 5p/CypB 的表达,对自身通路起到正反馈激活作用。

IL – 6 – STAT3 分子通路首先被发现在免疫系统中起调控 Th17 细胞、巨噬细胞以及树突状细胞的分化。随后研究发现,IL – 6 通过多条信号通路对肿瘤细胞的生长发挥促进作用。IL – 6 上调造成的 STAT3 激活能够上调 Cyclin D1、D2 和 B1,以及 c – Myc,并抑制 Cdk 抑制分子 P21 的表达,因而促进细胞进入细胞周期循环。IL – 6 也是细胞存活的重要调控分子,能够帮助肿瘤细胞逃逸应急和化疗药物造成的细胞死亡。IL – 6 激活的 STAT3 能够促进存活相关蛋白的表达,包括 Bcl – 2、Bcl – XL、Mcl – 1、Survivin 和 XIAP。这些蛋白的上调和持续激活的 STAT3 通常同肿瘤化疗耐药的机制有关。另外,IL – 6 通过增加端粒酶活性抑制细胞衰老，从而促进细胞生长。IL-6也能够通过介导EGF和HGF家族的相互作用来促进增殖。IL-11也通过类似的机制促进细胞增殖，抑制细胞凋亡。

IL-6还能够在多种肿瘤细胞中促进细胞转移和侵袭。JAK-STAT3信号通路的激活诱导产生基质金属蛋白酶（matrix metallo-proteinase，MMP）的MMP-2、MMP-7、MMP-9，这些蛋白能够降解细胞外基质，促进肿瘤侵袭。上皮间质转化（epithelial-mesenchymal transition，EMT）是机体发育过程中的正常生理现象，肿瘤侵袭入其他组织和血管中并形成远处转移的过程中也出现了EMT的现象。炎症是EMT的一个重要启动因子，IL-6也被发现在多种肿瘤细胞中够诱导EMT现象的发生。

IL-6能够在实体瘤中促进肿瘤血管生成。近期越来越多的证据表明IL-6信号通路的激活可能是VEGF-A抗体治疗癌症失败的原因之一。IL-6发挥促进血管生成的作用主要通过STAT3信号通路实现。后者的激活导致缺氧诱导因子1（Hypox-ia inducible factor-1，HIF-1）介导的VEGF-A的转录，同时也促进了内皮细胞增殖和迁移。HIF-1α同样被报道是STAT3的靶分子。IL-6还可能通过影响免疫细胞的表型，以增加血管生成因子的分泌来达到促进肿瘤细胞对抑制血管生成药物的耐受能力。对IL-6的靶向治疗能够抑制Notch配体Jagged-1的表达和卵巢癌细胞的血管微环境。在结肠癌患者中，血清中IL-6水平越高，肿瘤分期越差，转移性越强。

此外，IL-6还通过其他机制促进肿瘤转移。在IL-6表达较高的器官如脑、肺、肝、骨髓等部位，循环肿瘤细胞更趋向于定植和建立转移灶。例如，库普弗细胞中NF-κB的激活促进IL-6产生，后者进而促进肺转移癌细胞在肝脏的生长。人黑色素瘤细胞中STAT3的激活通过增加FGF、MMP-2、VEGF-A等促侵袭和血管生成分子的表达诱导肿瘤脑转移灶的形成和生长。此外，结肠癌患者循环中高水平的 IL‑6 同肝转移形成率相关。乳腺癌的骨转移也同上调的 IL‑6 表达和激活的 gp130‑STAT3 信号通路有关。

　　这些研究均表明 IL‑6 激活 STAT3 后，进一步通过下游癌基因的激活和抑癌基因的抑制，调控多种肿瘤的增殖、侵袭、转移、血管生成等表型。但是，肿瘤中 STAT3 一旦受到 IL‑6 刺激活化后，其状态长期处于持续激活的状态，即使去除 IL‑6 的刺激，这种持续激活的 STAT3 状态仍然不发生变化。这种现象的原因尚鲜有文献报道。在我们的研究中，我们发现的 CypB/STAT3/miR‑520d‑5p 反馈环路调控胃癌的模式可能有助于解释 STAT3 持续激活的机制。在正常胃癌组织中，miR‑520d‑5p 的表达相对较高，CypB 的表达较低，STAT3 通路处于不被激活的状态；在 Hp 感染的刺激下，巨噬细胞和胃上皮细胞产生 IL‑6，促进 JAK/STAT3 通路的激活，该通路能够抑制细胞中 miR‑520d‑5p 的转录及表达，导致 CypB 的表达增高，进一步促进了 STAT3 的磷酸化和入核，促进了细胞的恶性转化。

（李　铤　时永全）

参考文献

[1] Jemal A, Bray F, Center MM, et al. Global cancer statistics. CA‑Cancer J Clin, 2011, 61: 69‑90.

[2] Lertpiriyapong K, Whary MT, Muthupalani S, et al. Gastric colonisation with a restricted commensal microbiota replicates the promotion of neoplastic lesions by diverse intestinal microbiota in the Helicobacter pylori INS‑GAS mouse model of gastric carcinogenesis. Gut, 2014, 63: 54‑63.

[3] Taniguchi K, Karin M. IL‑6 and related cytokines as the critical lynchpins between inflammation and cancer. Semin Immunol, 2014, 26: 54‑74.

[4]　Li P, Shan JX, Chen XH, et al. Epigenetic silencing of microRNA-149 in cancer-associated fibroblasts mediates prostaglandin E2/interleukin-6 signaling in the tumor microenvironment. Cell Res, 2015, 25: 588-603.

[5]　Liao WC, Lin JT, Wu CY, et al. Serum interleukin-6 level but not genotype predicts survival after resection in stages Ⅱ and Ⅲ gastric carcinoma. Clin Cancer Res, 2008, 14: 428-434.

[6]　Lin MT, Lin BR, Chang CC, et al. IL-6 induces AGS gastric cancer cell invasion via activation of the c-Src/RhoA/ROCK signaling pathway. Int J Cancer, 2007, 120: 2600-2608.

[7]　Fichtner-Feigl S, Kesselring R, Strober W. Chronic inflammation and the development of malignancy in the GI tract. Trends Immunol, 2015, 36: 451-459.

[8]　Yu H, Pardoll D, Jove R. STATs in cancer inflammation and immunity: a leading role for STAT3. Nat Rev Cancer, 2009, 9: 798-809.

[9]　Yu H, Lee H, Herrmann A, et al. Revisiting STAT3 signalling in cancer: new and unexpected biological functions. Nat Rev Cancer, 2014, 14: 736-746.

[10]　Menheniott TR, Judd LM, Giraud AS. STAT3: a critical component in the response to Helicobacter pylori infection. Cell Microbiol, 2015, 17: 1570-1582.

[11]　Choi JW, Schroeder MA, Sarkaria JN, et al. Cyclophilin B supports Myc and mutant p53-dependent survival of glioblastoma multiforme cells. Cancer Res, 2014, 74: 484-496.

[12]　Bauer K, Kretzschmar AK, Cvijic H, et al. Cyclophilins contribute to Stat3 signaling and survival of multiple myeloma cells. Oncogene, 2009, 28: 2784-2795.

[13]　Kim Y, Jang M, Lim S, et al. Role of cyclophilin B in tumorigenesis and cisplatin resistance in hepatocellular carcinoma in humans. Hepatology, 2011, 54: 1661-1678.

[14]　Ray P, Rialon-Guevara KL, Veras E, et al. Comparing human pancreatic cell secretomes by in vitro aptamer selection identifies cyclophilin B as a candidate pancreatic cancer biomarker. J Clin Invest, 2012, 122:

1734 – 1741.

[15] Bartel DP. MicroRNAs: target recognition and regulatory functions. Cell, 2009, 136: 215 – 233.

[16] Lujambio A, Lowe SW. The microcosmos of cancer. Nature, 2012, 482: 347 – 355.

[17] Sitas F. Twenty five years since the first prospective study by Forman et al. (1991) on Helicobacter pylori and stomach cancer risk. Cancer Epidemiol, 2016, 41:159 – 164.

[18] Flisiak R, Horban A, Gallay P, et al. The cyclophilin inhibitor debio – 025 shows potent anti – hepatitis C effect in patients coinfected with hepatitis C and human immunodeficiency virus. Hepatology, 2008, 47: 817 – 826.

[19] Watashi K, Ishii N, Hijikata M, et al. Cyclophilin B is a functional regulator of hepatitis C virus RNA polymerase. Mol Cell, 2005, 19: 111 – 122.

[20] Choi JW, Sutor SL, Lindquist L, et al. Severe osteogenesis imperfecta in cyclophilin B – deficient mice. PLoS Genet, 2009, 5: e1000750.

[21] Fang F, Flegler AJ, Du P, et al. Expression of cyclophilin B is associated with malignant progression and regulation of genes implicated in the pathogenesis of breast cancer. Am J Pathol, 2009, 174: 297 – 308.

[22] Yan L, Yu J, Tan F, et al. SP1 – mediated microRNA – 520d – 5p suppresses tumor growth and metastasis in colorectal cancer by targeting CTHRC1. Am J Cancer Res, 2015, 5: 1447 – 1459.

[23] Tsukerman P, Yamin R, Seidel E, et al. MiR – 520d – 5p directly targets TWIST1 and downregulates the metastamiR miR – 10b. Oncotarget, 2014, 5: 12141 – 12150.

[24] Rokavec M, Oner MG, Li H, et al. IL – 6R/STAT3/miR – 34a feedback loop promotes EMT – mediated colorectal cancer invasion and metastasis. J Clin Invest, 2014, 124: 1853 – 1867.

[25] Rokavec M, Wu W, Luo JL. IL6 – mediated suppression of miR – 200c directs constitutive activation of inflammatory signaling circuit driving transformation and tumorigenesis. Mol Cell, 2012, 45: 777 – 789.

[26] Shen S, Guo X, Yan H, et al. A miR – 130a – YAP positive feedback loop

promotes organ size and tumorigenesis. Cell Res, 2015, 25: 997 – 1012.

[27] Zhao XD, Lu YY, Guo H, et al. MicroRNA – 7/NF – kappaB signaling regulatory feedback circuit regulates gastric carcinogenesis. J Cell Biol, 2015, 210: 613 – 627.

[28] de Sablet T, Piazuelo MB, Shaffer CL, et al. Phylogeographic origin of Helicobacter pylori is a determinant of gastric cancer risk. Gut, 2011, 60: 1189 – 1195.

[29] Peek RM Jr, Fiske C, Wilson KT. Role of innate immunity in Helicobacter pylori – induced gastric malignancy. Physiol Rev, 2010, 90: 831 – 858.

[30] Wilson KT, Crabtree JE. Immunology of Helicobacter pylori: insights into the failure of the immune response and perspectives on vaccine studies. Gastroenterology, 2007, 133: 288 – 308.

[31] Augusto AC, Miguel F, Mendonca S, et al. Oxidative stress expression status associated to Helicobacter pylori virulence in gastric diseases. Clin Biochem, 2007, 40: 615 – 622.

[32] Chaturvedi R, de Sablet T, Coburn LA, et al. Arginine and polyamines in Helicobacter pylori – induced immune dysregulation and gastric carcinogenesis. Amino Acids, 2012, 42: 627 – 640.

[33] Hardbower DM, Peek RM, Wilson KT. At the Bench: Helicobacter pylori, dysregulated host responses, DNA damage, and gastric cancer. J Leukoc Biol, 2014, 96: 201 – 212.

[34] Lin WC, Tsai HF, Kuo SH, et al. Translocation of Helicobacter pylori CagA into Human B lymphocytes, the origin of mucosa – associated lymphoid tissue lymphoma. Cancer Res, 2010, 70: 5740 – 5748.

[35] Chaturvedi R, Asim M, Romero – Gallo J, et al. Spermine Oxidase Mediates the Gastric Cancer Risk Associated With Helicobacter pylori CagA. Gastroenterology, 2011, 141: 1696 – 708. e2.

[36] Raju D, Hussey S, Ang M, et al. Vacuolating cytotoxin and variants in Atg16L1 that disrupt autophagy promote Helicobacter pylori infection in humans. Gastroenterology, 2012, 142: 1160 – 1171.

[37] Kim JM, Kim JS, Lee JY, et al. Vacuolating cytotoxin in Helicobacter py-

lori water – soluble proteins upregulates chemokine expression in human e-osinophils via Ca^{2+} influx, mitochondrial reactive oxygen intermediates, and NF – kappaB activation. Infect Immun, 2007, 75: 3373 – 3381.

[38] Eruslanov E, Kusmartsev S. Identification of ROS using oxidized DCFDA and flow – cytometry. Methods Mol Biol, 2010, 594: 57 – 72.

[39] Tsugawa H, Suzuki H, Saya H, et al. Reactive oxygen species – induced autophagic degradation of Helicobacter pylori CagA is specifically suppressed in cancer stem – like cells. Cell Host Microbe, 2012, 12: 764 – 777.

[40] Wang G, Hong Y, Olczak A, et al. Dual Roles of Helicobacter pylori NapA in Inducing and Combating Oxidative Stress. Infect Immun, 2006, 74: 6839 – 6846.

[41] Uberti AF, Olivera – Severo D, Wassermann GE, et al. Pro – inflammatory properties and neutrophil activation by Helicobacter pylori urease. Toxicon, 2013, 69: 240 – 249.

[42] Gong M, Ling SSM, Lui SY, et al. Helicobacter pylori γ – Glutamyl Transpeptidase Is a Pathogenic Factor in the Development of Peptic Ulcer Disease. Gastroenterology, 2010, 139: 564 – 573.

[43] Eftang LL, Esbensen Y, Tannæs TM, et al. Interleukin – 8 is the single most up – regulated gene in whole genome profiling of H. pylori exposed gastric epithelial cells. BMC Microbiol, 2012, 12: 9.

[44] Asfaha S, Dubeykovskiy AN, Tomita H, et al. Mice That Express Human Interleukin – 8 Have Increased Mobilization of Immature Myeloid Cells, Which Exacerbates Inflammation and Accelerates Colon Carcinogenesis. Gastroenterology, 2013, 144: 155 – 166.

[45] Li M, Zhang Y, Feurino LW, et al. Interleukin – 8 increases vascular endothelial growth factor and neuropilin expression and stimulates ERK activation in human pancreatic cancer. Cancer Sci, 2008, 99: 733 – 737.

[46] Wang Y, Xu RC, Zhang XL, et al. Interleukin – 8 secretion by ovarian cancer cells increases anchorage – independent growth, proliferation, angiogenic potential, adhesion and invasion. Cytokine, 2012, 59: 145 – 155.

[47] Sugimoto M, Ohno T, Graham DY, et al. Helicobacter pylori outer mem-

brane proteins on gastric mucosal interleukin 6 and 11 expression in Mongolian gerbils. J　Gastroenterol Hepatol, 2011, 26: 1677 – 1684.

[48] Nakagawa H, Tamura T, Mitsuda Y, et al. Significant association between serum interleukin – 6 and Helicobacter pylori antibody levels among H. pylori – positive Japanese adults. Mediat Inflamm, 2013, 2013: 142358.

[49] Bronte – Tinkew DM, Terebiznik M, Franco A, et al. Helicobacter pylori cytotoxin – associated gene A activates the signal transducer and activator of transcription 3 pathway in vitro and in vivo. Cancer Res, 2009, 69: 632 – 639.

[50] Garbers C, Hermanns HM, Schaper F, et al. Plasticity and cross – talk of Interleukin 6 – type cytokines. Cytokine Growth Factor Rev, 2012, 23: 85 – 97.

[51] Kishimoto T. IL – 6: from its discovery to clinical applications. Int Immunol, 2010, 22: 347 – 352.

[52] Taniguchi K, Karin M. IL – 6 and related cytokines as the critical lynchpins between inflammation and cancer. Semin Immunol, 2014, 26: 54 – 74.

[53] Howlett M, Menheniott TR, Judd LM, et al. Cytokine signalling via gp130 in gastric cancer. Biochim Biophys Acta, 2009, 1793: 1623 – 1633.

[54] Rose – John S, Mitsuyama K, Matsumoto S, et al. Interleukin – 6 trans – signaling and colonic cancer associated with inflammatory bowel disease. Curr Pharm Des, 2009, 15: 2095 – 2103.

[55] Scheller J, Chalaris A, Schmidt – Arras D, et al. The pro – and anti – inflammatory properties of the cytokine interleukin – 6. Biochim Biophys Acta, 2011, 1813: 878 – 888.

[56] Yoshimura A, Yasukawa H. JAK's SOCS: a mechanism of inhibition. Immunity, 2012, 36: 157 – 159.

[57] Yoshimura A, Naka T, Kubo M. SOCS proteins, cytokine signalling and immune regulation. Nat Rev Immunol, 2007, 7: 454 – 465.

[58] Wang Y, van Boxel – Dezaire AHH, Cheon H, et al. STAT3 activation in response to IL – 6 is prolonged by the binding of IL – 6 receptor to EGF

receptor. Proc Natl Acad Sci, 2013, 110: 16975 – 16980.

[59] Ara T, DeClerck YA. Interleukin – 6 in bone metastasis and cancer progression. Eur J Cancer, 2010, 46: 1223 – 1231.

[60] Grivennikov SI, Karin M. Inflammatory cytokines in cancer: tumour necrosis factor and interleukin 6 take the stage. Ann Rheum Dis, 2011, 70: i104 – 108.

[61] Guo Y, Xu F, Lu T, et al. Interleukin – 6 signaling pathway in targeted therapy for cancer. Cancer Treat Rev, 2012, 38: 904 – 910.

[62] Poncet N, Guillaume J, Mouchiroud G. Epidermal growth factor receptor transactivation is implicated in IL – 6 – induced proliferation and ERK1/2 activation in non – transformed prostate epithelial cells. Cell Signal, 2011, 23: 572 – 578.

[63] Hov H, Tian E, Holien T, et al. c – Met signaling promotes IL – 6 – induced myeloma cell proliferation. Eur J Haematol, 2009, 82: 277 – 287.

[64] Garbers C, Scheller J. Interleukin – 6 and interleukin – 11: same same but different. Biol Chem, 2013, 394: 1145 – 1161.

[65] Putoczki T, Ernst M. More than a sidekick: the IL – 6 family cytokine IL – 11 links inflammation to cancer. J Leukoc Biol, 2010, 88: 1109 – 1117.

[66] Walter M, Liang S, Ghosh S, et al. Interleukin 6 secreted from adipose stromal cells promotes migration and invasion of breast cancer cells. Oncogene, 2009, 28: 2745 – 2755.

[67] Foran E, Garrity – Park MM, Mureau C, et al. Upregulation of DNA methyltransferase – mediated gene silencing, anchorage – i ndependent growth, and migration of colon cancer cells by interleukin – 6. Mol Cancer Res, 2010, 8: 471 – 481.

[68] Mano Y, Aishima S, Fujita N, et al. Tumor – associated macrophage promotes tumor progression via STAT3 signaling in hepatocellular carcinoma. Pathobiology, 2013, 80: 146 – 154.

[69] Lay V, Yap J, Sonderegger S, et al. Interleukin 11 regulates endometrial cancer cell adhesion and migration via STAT3. Int J Oncol, 2012, 41: 759 – 764.

[70] Nakayama T, Yoshizaki A, Izumida S, et al. Expression of interleukin –

11（IL－11）and IL－11 receptor α in human gastric carcinoma and IL－11 upregulates the invasive activity of human gastric carcinoma cells. Int J Oncol, 2007, 30: 825－833.

[71]　Nieto MA. Epithelial plasticity: a common theme in embryonic and cancer cells. Science, 2013, 342: 1234850.

[72]　De Craene B, Berx G. Regulatory networks defining EMT during cancer initiation and progression. Nat Rev Cancer, 2013, 13: 97－110.

[73]　Tsai JH, Yang J. Epithelial－mesenchymal plasticity in carcinoma metastasis. Genes Dev, 2013, 27: 2192－2206.

[74]　Tam WL, Weinberg RA. The epigenetics of epithelial－mesenchymal plasticity in cancer. Nat Med, 2013, 19: 1438－1449.

[75]　Creighton CJ, Gibbons DL, Kurie JM. The role of epithelial－mesenchymal transition programming in invasion and metastasis: a clinical perspective. Cancer Manag Res, 2013, 5: 187－195.

[76]　Sullivan NJ, Sasser AK, Axel AE, et al. Interleukin－6 induces an epithelial－mesenchymal transition phenotype in human breast cancer cells. Oncogene, 2009, 28: 2940－2947.

[77]　Huang C, Yang G, Jiang T, et al. The effects and mechanisms of blockage of STAT3 signaling pathway on IL－6 inducing EMT in human pancreatic cancer cells in vitro. Neoplasma, 2011, 58: 396－405.

[78]　Yadav A, Kumar B, Datta J, et al. IL－6 promotes head and neck tumor metastasis by inducing epithelial－mesenchymal transition via the JAK－STAT3－SNAIL signaling pathway. Mol Cancer Res, 2011, 9: 1658－1667.

[79]　Middleton K, Jones J, Lwin Z, et al. Interleukin－6: An angiogenic target in solid tumours. Crit Rev Oncol Hematol, 2014, 89: 129－139.

[80]　Dang Eric V, Barbi J, Yang H－Y, et al. Control of TH17/Treg balance by hypoxia－inducible factor 1. Cell, 2011, 146: 772－784.

[81]　Coward J, Kulbe H, Chakravarty P, et al. Interleukin－6 as a therapeutic target in human ovarian cancer. Clin Cancer Res, 2011, 17: 6083－6096.

[82]　Eldesoky A, Shouma A, Mosaad Y, et al. Clinical relevance of serum vascular endothelial growth factor and interleukin－6 in patients with

colorectal cancer. Saudi J Gastroenterol, 2011, 17: 170 – 173.

[83] Maeda S, Hikiba Y, Sakamoto K, et al. Ikappa B kinasebeta/nuclear factor – kappaB activation controls the development of liver metastasis by way of interleukin – 6 expression. Hepatology, 2009, 50: 1851 – 1860.

[84] Ren L, Wang X, Dong Z, et al. Bone metastasis from breast cancer involves elevated IL – 11 expression and the gp130/STAT3 pathway. Med Oncol, 2013, 30: 634.

[85] McCoy CE. The role of miRNAs in cytokine signaling. Front Biosci, 2011, 16: 2161.

[86] Cao Q, Li YY, He WF, et al. Interplay between microRNAs and the STAT3 signaling pathway in human cancers. Physiol Genomics, 2013, 45: 1206 – 1214.

[87] Loffler D, Brocke – Heidrich K, Pfeifer G, et al. Interleukin – 6 dependent survival of multiple myeloma cells involves the Stat3 – mediated induction of microRNA – 21 through a highly conserved enhancer. Blood, 2007, 110: 1330 – 1333.

[88] Meng F, Henson R, Wehbe – Janek H, et al. The MicroRNA let – 7a modulates interleukin – 6 – dependent STAT – 3 survival signaling in malignant human cholangiocytes. J Biol Chem, 2007, 282: 8256 – 8264.

[89] Haider KH, Idris NM, Kim HW, et al. MicroRNA – 21 is a key determinant in IL – 11/Stat3 anti – apoptotic signalling pathway in preconditioning of skeletal myoblasts. Cardiovasc Res, 2010, 88: 168 – 178.

[90] Iliopoulos D, Hirsch HA, Struhl K. An epigenetic switch involving NF – kappaB, Lin28, Let – 7 MicroRNA, and IL6 links inflammation to cell transformation. Cell, 2009, 139: 693 – 706.

[91] Pichiorri F, Suh SS, Ladetto M, et al. MicroRNAs regulate critical genes associated with multiple myeloma pathogenesis. Proc Natl Acad Sci, 2008, 105: 12885 – 12890.

[92] Pollari S, Leivonen SK, Perala M, et al. Identification of microRNAs inhibiting TGF – beta – induced IL – 11 production in bone metastatic breast cancer cells. PloS One, 2012, 7: e37361.

[93] Yang X, Liang L, Zhang XF, et al. MicroRNA-26a suppresses tumor growth and metastasis of human hepatocellular carcinoma by targeting interleukin-6-Stat3 pathway. Hepatology, 2013, 58:158-70.

[94] He Y, Sun X, Huang C, et al. MiR-146a regulates IL-6 production in lipopolysaccharide-induced RAW264. 7 macrophage cells by inhibiting Notch1. Inflammation, 2014, 37: 71-82.

[95] Bockhorn J, Dalton R, Nwachukwu C, et al. MicroRNA-30c inhibits human breast tumour chemotherapy resistance by regulating TWF1 and IL-11. Nat Commun, 2013, 4: 1393.

[96] Jin D-Y, Collins AS, McCoy CE, et al. miR-19a: An effective regulator of SOCS3 and enhancer of JAK-STAT signalling. PloS One, 2013, 8: e69090.

[97] Liao WC, Lin JT, Wu CY, et al. Serum Interleukin-6 level but not genotype predicts survival after resection in stages Ⅱ and Ⅲ gastric carcinoma. Clin Cancer Res, 2008, 14: 428-434.

[98] Jackson CB, Judd LM, Menheniott TR, et al. Augmented gp130-mediated cytokine signalling accompanies human gastric cancer progression. J Pathol, 2007, 213: 140-151.

[99] Ernst M, Najdovska M, Grail D, et al. STAT3 and STAT1 mediate IL-11-dependent and inflammation-associated gastric tumorigenesis in gp130 receptor mutant mice. J Clin Invest, 2008, 118: 1727-1738.

[100] Howlett M, Giraud AS, Lescesen H, et al. The interleukin-6 family cytokine interleukin-11 regulates homeostatic epithelial cell turnover and promotes gastric tumor development. Gastroenterology, 2009, 136: 967-977. e3.

[101] Putoczki Tracy L, Thiem S, Loving A, et al. Interleukin-11 is the dominant IL-6 family cytokine during gastrointestinal tumorigenesis and can be targeted therapeutically. Cancer Cell, 2013, 24: 257-271.

[102] Algül H, Kinoshita H, Hirata Y, et al. Interleukin-6 mediates epithelial-stromal interactions and promotes gastric tumorigenesis. PloS One, 2013, 8: e60914.

[103] Correa P, Houghton J. Carcinogenesis of Helicobacter pylori. Gastroenterology, 2007, 133: 659 –672.

[104] Takaishi S, Tu S, Dubeykovskaya ZA, et al. Gastrin is an essential co-
factor for helicobacter – associated gastric corpus carcinogenesis in
C57BL/6 mice. Am J Pathol, 2009, 175: 365 –375.

[105] Judd LM, Bredin K, Kalantzis A, et al. STAT3 activation regulates
growth, inflammation, and vascularization in a mouse model of gastric
tumorigenesis. Gastroenterology, 2006, 131: 1073 –1085.

[106] Tu S, Bhagat G, Cui G, et al. Overexpression of interleukin – 1β induces gastric inflammation and cancer and mobilizes myeloid – derived
suppressor cells in mice. Cancer Cell, 2011, 19: 154.

[107] Howlett M, Chalinor HV, Buzzelli JN, et al. IL – 11 is a parietal cell
cytokine that induces atrophic gastritis. Gut, 2011, 61: 1398 –1409.

[108] Poppe M, Feller SM, Römer G, et al. Phosphorylation of Helicobacter
pylori CagA by c – Abl leads to cell motility. Oncogene, 2006, 26:
3462 –3472.

[109] Saadat I, Higashi H, Obuse C, et al. Helicobacter pylori CagA targets
PAR1/MARK kinase to disrupt epithelial cell polarity. Nature, 2007,
447: 330 –333.

[110] Lee KS, Kalantzis A, Jackson CB, et al. Helicobacter pylori CagA triggers expression of the bactericidal lectin REG3gamma via gastric STAT3
activation. PloS One, 2012, 7: e30786.

[111] Lee IO, Kim JH, Choi YJ, et al. Helicobacter pylori CagA phosphorylation status determines the gp130 – activated SHP2/ERK and JAK/STAT
signal transduction pathways in gastric epithelial cells. J Biol Chem,
2010, 285: 16042 –16050.

[112] Matsumoto A, Isomoto H, Nakayama M, et al. Helicobacter pylori VacA
reduces the cellular expression of STAT3 and pro – survival Bcl – 2 family proteins, Bcl – 2 and Bcl – XL, leading to apoptosis in gastric epithelial cells. Dig Dis Sci, 2010, 56: 999 –1006.

[113] Giraud AS, Menheniott TR, Judd LM. Targeting STAT3 in gastric canc-

er. Expert Opin Ther Targets, 2012, 16: 889 - 901.

[114] Sneddon JB, Zhen HH, Montgomery K, et al. Bone morphogenetic protein antagonist gremlin 1 is widely expressed by cancer - associated stromal cells and can promote tumor cell proliferation. Proc Natl Acad Sci, 2006, 103: 14842 - 14847.

[115] Namkoong H, Shin SM, Kim HK, et al. The bone morphogenetic protein antagonist gremlin 1 is overexpressed in human cancers and interacts with YWHAH protein. BMC Cancer, 2006, 6: 74.

[116] Petsko GA, Davis TL, Walker JR, et al. Structural and biochemical characterization of the human cyclophilin family of peptidyl - prolyl isomerases. PLoS Biol, 2010, 8: e1000439.

[117] Nigro P, Pompilio G, Capogrossi MC. Cyclophilin A: a key player for human disease. Cell Death Dis, 2013, 4: e888.

[118] Hoffmann H, Schiene - Fischer C. Functional aspects of extracellular cyclophilins. Biol Chem, 2014, 395: 721 - 735.

[119] Gallay PA. Cyclophilin inhibitors: a novel class of promising host - targeting anti - HCV agents. Immunol Res, 2011, 52: 200 - 210.

[120] Wang L, Wang CH, Jia JF, et al. Contribution of cyclophilin A to the regulation of inflammatory processes in rheumatoid arthritis. J Clin Immunol, 2009, 30: 24 - 33.

[121] Yang Y, Lu N, Zhou J, et al. Cyclophilin A up - regulates MMP - 9 expression and adhesion of monocytes/macrophages via CD147 signalling pathway in rheumatoid arthritis. Rheumatology, 2008, 47:1299 - 1310.

[122] Satoh K, Nigro P, Matoba T, et al. Cyclophilin A enhances vascular oxidative stress and the development of angiotensin II - induced aortic aneurysms. Nat Med, 2009, 15: 649 - 656.

[123] Elrod JW, Molkentin JD. Physiologic functions of cyclophilin D and the mitochondrial permeability transition pore. Circ J, 2013, 77: 1111 - 1122.

[124] Rasola A, Bernardi P. Mitochondrial permeability transition in Ca^{2+} - dependent apoptosis and necrosis. Cell Calcium, 2011, 50: 222 - 233.

[125] Linkermann A, Green DR. Necroptosis. N Engl J Med, 2014, 370: 455-465.

[126] Linkermann A, Brasen JH, Darding M, et al. Two independent pathways of regulated necrosis mediate ischemia - reperfusion injury. Proc Natl Acad Sci, 2013, 110: 12024-12029.

[127] Ray P, Rialon - Guevara KL, Veras E, et al. Comparing human pancreatic cell secretomes by in vitro aptamer selection identifies cyclophilin B as a candidate pancreatic cancer biomarker. J Clin Invest, 2012, 122: 1734-1741.

[128] Fang F, Flegler AJ, Du P, et al. Expression of cyclophilin B is associated with malignant progression and regulation of genes implicated in the pathogenesis of breast cancer. Am J Pathol, 2009, 174: 297-308.

[129] Fang F, Zheng J, Galbaugh TL, et al. Cyclophilin B as a co - regulator of prolactin - induced gene expression and function in breast cancer cells. J Mol Endocrinol, 2010, 44: 319-329.

[130] Williams PD, Owens CR, Dziegielewski J, et al. Cyclophilin B expression is associated with in vitro radioresistance and clinical outcome after radiotherapy. Neoplasia, 2011, 13: 1122-1131.

[131] Kim K, Kim H, Jeong K, et al. Release of overexpressed CypB activates ERK signaling through CD147 binding for hepatoma cell resistance to oxidative stress. Apoptosis, 2012, 17: 784-796.

[132] Jeong K, Kim H, Kim K, et al. Cyclophilin B is involved in p300 - mediated degradation of CHOP in tumor cell adaptation to hypoxia. Cell Death Differ, 2014, 21: 438-450.

[133] Li X, Zhang Y, Zhang Y, et al. Survival prediction of gastric cancer by a seven - microRNA signature. Gut, 2009, 59: 579-585.

[134] Godlewski J, Nowicki MO, Bronisz A, et al. Targeting of the Bmi - 1 oncogene/stem cell renewal factor by microRNA - 128 inhibits glioma proliferation and self - renewal. Cancer Res, 2008, 68: 9125-9130.

[135] Keklikoglou I, Koerner C, Schmidt C, et al. MicroRNA - 520/373 family functions as a tumor suppressor in estrogen receptor negative breast

cancer by targeting NF − kappaB and TGF − beta signaling pathways. Oncogene, 2012, 31: 4150 −4163.

[136] Park YY, Kim SB, Han HD, et al. Tat − activating regulatory DNA − binding protein regulates glycolysis in hepatocellular carcinoma by regulating the platelet isoform of phosphofructokinase through microRNA 520. Hepatology, 2013, 58: 182 − 191.

[137] Jiang H, Dong Q, Luo X, et al. The monoclonal antibody CH12 augments 5 − fluorouracil − induced growth suppression of hepatocellular carcinoma xenografts expressing epidermal growth factor receptor variant Ⅲ. Cancer Lett, 2014, 342: 113 − 120.

第二章

分泌型糖蛋白的糖基化修饰
与胃癌多药耐药

　　近年来，人们发现肿瘤细胞分泌蛋白作为重要的细胞外因素也参与了对肿瘤耐药性的调节。研究发现，肿瘤细胞分泌蛋白的种类和数量在其对化疗药物产生耐药以后发生了显著的变化。相当数量的肿瘤细胞分泌蛋白在分泌到胞外之前都会经历糖基化修饰。研究人员发现糖蛋白糖基化修饰的改变可以极大地影响肿瘤对化疗药物的敏感性，对肿瘤多药耐药的形成起着至关重要的作用。然而，既往的研究极少关注肿瘤细胞分泌蛋白糖基化修饰尤其是位点特异性糖基化修饰在肿瘤多药耐药中的作用。因此，对耐药过程中胃癌细胞分泌蛋白糖基化修饰特别是位点特异性糖基化修饰的解析，有助于我们得到与胃癌多药耐药相关的特定糖型以及异常糖基化的糖蛋白，从而更好地阐明胃癌多药耐药的发生机制，并为胃癌耐药的预测和逆转找出可能的分子标志物。

一、肿瘤微环境与肿瘤耐药

　　肿瘤耐药的产生是包括细胞外因素在内的多种因素综合作用的结果，而之前的研究大都着眼于肿瘤细胞内因素在肿瘤多药耐药中的作用，忽视了细胞外因素在耐药产生中的重要作用。现在，人们越来越清楚地认识到了肿瘤细胞外因素对肿瘤耐药的重要意义，发现肿瘤微环境中的巨噬细胞、成纤维细胞、淋巴细胞以及细胞外基质等可以通过直接或间接的细胞间相互作用来影响肿瘤细胞对化疗药物的敏感性。对胃癌等实体肿瘤而言，肿瘤微环境主要包括细胞外基质（extracellular matrix，ECM）、肿瘤相关成纤维细胞（cancer - associated fibroblasts，CAFs）和肿瘤相关巨噬细胞（tumor - associated macrophages，TAMs）等免疫细胞、血管，以及这些相关细胞分泌的细胞因子等（图 2 - 1）。

　　肿瘤微环境中的多种细胞及其分泌的细胞因子可以促进肿瘤的生长、血管生成和侵袭等，因此肿瘤微环境在肿瘤的发生、发展以及转移中发挥着重要的作用。此外，肿瘤微环境中的细胞外基质、部分基质细胞可以通过与肿瘤细胞之间直接或间接的相互作用来抑制药物诱导的细胞死亡，促进肿瘤细胞在药物应激下的存活，进而参与调节肿瘤对化疗药物的敏感性（图 2 - 2）。近年来，研究人员已陆续发现了微环境中的成纤维细胞、巨噬细胞、细胞外基质、细胞因子以及肿瘤细胞自分泌蛋白在肿瘤耐药产生中的重要意义，下面我们将从这几个方面详细论述肿瘤微环境对肿瘤耐药的调节作用。

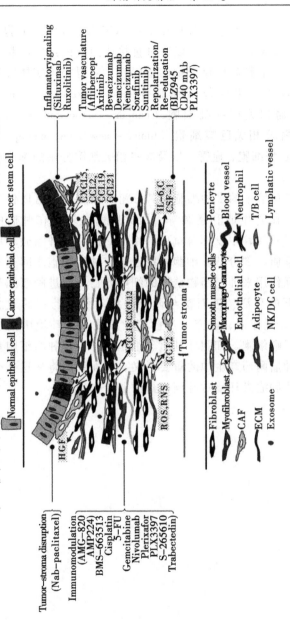

图2-1　肿瘤微环境的主要成分

（引自Cancer Lett, 2015, 380:205-215）

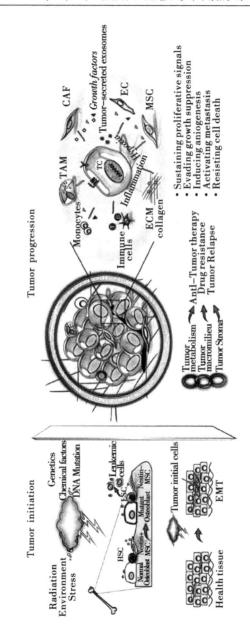

图2-2　肿瘤微环境参与肿瘤的发生、发展和耐药
（引自Cancer Lett, 2015, 368: 7-13）

1. 肿瘤相关成纤维细胞

肿瘤相关成纤维细胞可以通过多种途径促进肿瘤耐药的发生。实体瘤中的成纤维细胞不同于体内正常的成纤维细胞，其在肿瘤内部发挥着不同的功能。实体瘤中定植的成纤维细胞在多种细胞因子如成纤维细胞生长因子（fibroblast growth factor，FGF）、单核细胞趋化蛋白 1（monocyte chemotactic protein 1，MCP - 1）、血小板源性生长因子（platelet - derived growth factor，PDGF）、组织金属蛋白酶抑制剂 1（tissue inhibitor of metalloproteinase 1，TIMP - 1）和转化生长因子 β（transforming growth factor β，TGF - β）等的作用下转化为肿瘤相关成纤维细胞。这些成纤维细胞不仅参与构成实体瘤的骨架，而且能够调控肿瘤细胞对化疗药物的敏感性。研究表明，在化疗药物的作用下，肿瘤相关成纤维细胞活化、增殖，并且通过 β1/FAK/Src 和 ERK/MAPK 途径促进黑色素瘤细胞耐药的产生。此外，人们发现化疗药物在杀伤前列腺癌细胞的同时，对微环境中的成纤维细胞也造成了损伤；受损的成纤维细胞发生损伤修复反应，细胞中 NF - κB 信号被激活，进而分泌 WNT16B，通过经典的 Wnt/β - catenin 信号通路促进癌细胞的增殖以及 EMT 的发生（上皮间质转化，epithelial to mesenchymal transition），从而使得前列腺癌细胞对化疗药物产生抵抗（图2 - 3）。

2. 肿瘤相关巨噬细胞

研究表明，肿瘤相关巨噬细胞可以介导肿瘤细胞对多种化疗药物的耐药。巨噬细胞可以上调胰腺导管癌细胞中胞嘧啶核苷脱氨酶的表达，进而使吉西他滨在胰腺癌细胞中失活，从而介导胰腺导管癌细胞对吉西他滨耐药。此外，在乳腺癌中，肿瘤相关巨噬细胞可以通过分泌 IL - 10，激活癌细胞中 Bcl - 2、STAT3 信号途径，进而介导乳腺癌中紫杉醇耐药的产生。

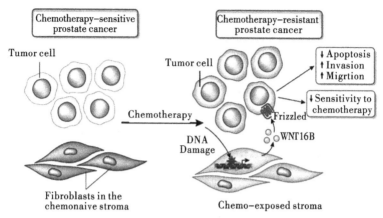

图 2 - 3　成纤维细胞促进前列腺癌细胞耐药的分子机制
（引自 Nat Med, 2012, 18: 1359 - 1368)

3. 细胞外基质

肿瘤细胞与细胞外基质的黏附可以介导其对化疗药物的耐药。细胞外基质由肿瘤微环境中的多种细胞生成，不仅为肿瘤细胞的生长提供纤维支架，而且参与调节肿瘤细胞的活性。研究发现，乳腺癌细胞黏附于细胞外基质后其极性以及细胞内 NF - κB 的活性发生改变，进而使得自身对药物诱导的凋亡发生抵抗，从而产生耐药。细胞黏附介导的耐药主要依赖于肿瘤细胞表面整联蛋白（integrin）与细胞外基质的相互作用。整联蛋白是细胞表面重要的黏附分子，与细胞外基质相互作用后可以调节肿瘤细胞内 PI3K/AKT，ERK 和 NF - κB 信号通路，从而抑制药物诱导的细胞凋亡，促进肿瘤细胞的存活。

4. 细胞因子

肿瘤微环境中各类基质细胞分泌的细胞因子可以激活肿瘤细胞的多种存活信号通路，继而促进肿瘤细胞耐药的发生。例如，肿瘤微环境中浸润的辅助性 T 细胞 17（Th17）可以通过分泌白介素 17（IL - 17）来介导肿瘤细胞对血管内皮生长因子单

克隆抗体 （VEGF monoclonal antibody） 的耐药。此外，研究人员发现，当基质细胞和黑色素瘤细胞共培养时基质细胞分泌的肝细胞生长因子 （hepatocyte growth factor，HGF） 可以激活肿瘤细胞表面的 HGF 受体，随后激活 MAPK 以及 PI3K/AKT 信号通路，进而介导黑色素瘤细胞对 RAF 抑制剂的耐受。

5. 肿瘤细胞自分泌因子

广义上讲，肿瘤细胞自分泌因子也是肿瘤微环境的重要组成部分，同时也参与了肿瘤耐药的产生。研究发现，BRAF、ALK 或 EGFR 激酶抑制剂用于人黑色素瘤和肺腺癌后可以诱导肿瘤细胞分泌一系列分子，这一药物诱导的肿瘤细胞分泌组可以刺激耐药细胞的增殖和播散，并且能够促进药敏细胞的存活。此外，人们发现来自耐药肿瘤细胞的胞外囊泡 （extracellular vesicles） 可使得药敏的肿瘤细胞对化疗药物产生抵抗。分泌型聚集素 （secreted clusterin，sCLU） 已被报道参与多种肿瘤耐药的产生，如骨肉瘤、肝细胞癌等。分泌型 sonic hedgehog 抑制药物诱导的细胞凋亡，参与多发性骨髓瘤多药耐药的产生。就胃癌而言，分泌型糖蛋白 WNT6 可以促进胃癌多药耐药的发生，VEGF – C 的分泌参与调节了胃癌对顺铂的抵抗。更重要的是，在蛋白组学技术的帮助下，人们发现胃癌耐药细胞系与药敏细胞系的分泌蛋白组之间存在着显著的差异。

二、蛋白糖基化修饰与肿瘤耐药

（一） 蛋白糖基化修饰概况

糖基化修饰是哺乳动物体内一种最普遍、最重要的蛋白翻译后修饰（post - translational modifications, PTMs），研究发现人体内一半以上的蛋白都会经历糖基化修饰，它对蛋白质的构象、结构和功能的发挥有着重要的作用，参与多种重要的细胞和分子生物学进程如细胞黏附、蛋白转运、受体激活和信号转导等。糖基化修饰是指将糖类化合物通过糖苷键连接到蛋白、多糖或脂类分子的复杂的酶促反应过程。根据与糖苷配基的连接特征的不同，可将糖缀合物分为多个类型（图 2 - 4），如 N - 多聚糖、O - 多聚糖、鞘糖脂和黏多糖等。就糖蛋白而言，根据糖链所连接的肽段序列和连接方式的不同可将蛋白质的糖基化分为 N - 糖基化、O - 糖基化、C - 糖基化和糖基化磷脂酰肌醇锚（GPI - anchored）等。N - 糖基化是指糖链连接在多肽序列中的天冬酰胺残基（asparagine, Asn）侧链上，并且其糖基化位点所在序列符合 NXS/T（X 是除脯氨酸外的任意氨基酸，S 为丝氨酸，T 为苏氨酸）；O - 糖基化是指糖链连接在多肽序列的丝氨酸（serine, Ser）或苏氨酸（threonine, Thr）残基侧链上，O - 糖基化的位点序列比较广泛；C - 糖基化是指糖链连接在肽段序列的半胱氨酸（cysteine, Cys）残基侧链上；糖基化磷脂酰肌醇锚是指蛋白质通过肽链的 C 端共价连接糖基化磷脂酰肌醇，并通过糖基化磷脂酰肌醇锚定在细胞膜上。不同种类的糖基化发挥着不同的功能，现阶段我们主要关注蛋白质的 N - 糖基化修饰。N - 糖基化的糖链一般由一个五碳糖核心和若干糖单元组成，大体上可分为高甘露糖型、复合型和杂合型三类（图 2 - 5），其组成有着特定的规律。

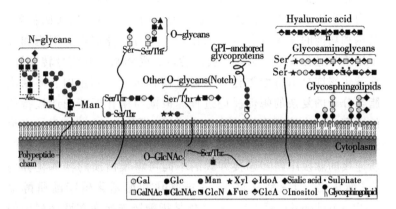

图 2 - 4　人体内糖缀合物的主要类别

（引自 Nat Rev Cancer, 2015, 15：540 - 555）

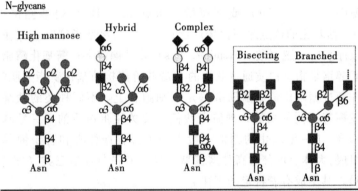

图 2 - 5　人体内 N - 糖基化的分类

（引自 Trends Mol Med, 2013, 19：664 - 676）

（二）蛋白糖基化修饰与肿瘤

蛋白的糖基化修饰参与肿瘤形成过程中众多重要的生物学进程如炎症、免疫监视、细胞间黏附、细胞与基质的相互作用、细胞内及细胞间的信号转导和细胞的代谢等，对肿瘤的发生、发展有着重要的调节作用（图 2-6）。因此，深入解析蛋白的糖基化修饰对阐明肿瘤的形成机制具有十分重要的意义。

糖蛋白 E-cadherin（epithelial cadherin，上皮细胞钙黏蛋白）是重要的细胞黏附分子，其功能的正常发挥对介导肿瘤细胞间黏附有着重要的意义。研究发现，胃癌细胞中 N-乙酰葡糖胺转移酶 V（N-acetylglucosaminyl transferase-V，GnT-V）的表达升高，引起了 E-cadherin 的糖基化修饰发生异常，进而干扰了细胞间的正常黏附，导致肿瘤的侵袭和转移；高表达 GnT-V 的胃癌细胞在小鼠肿瘤模型中的转移能力显著升高。此外，研究人员发现干扰 E-cadherin 的糖基化会影响其正常表达，例如，抑制 E-cadherin 在位点 Asn633 处的糖基化会影响 E-cadherin 的表达水平，导致 E-cadherin 通过内质网途径发生降解。

整联蛋白（integrin）是介导肿瘤细胞与细胞外基质相互作用的关键分子，在肿瘤的侵袭和转移中有着重要的作用。研究报道，整联蛋白的糖基化修饰能够影响其功能的正常发挥，并促进肿瘤的发生和转移。就胃癌而言，GnT-V 的过表达通过影响整联蛋白的糖基化修饰，从而促进细胞的迁移。然而，与 GnT-V 的作用相反，胃癌中 GnT-Ⅲ 的表达能够通过影响 GnT-V 对整联蛋白的糖基化修饰来抑制整联蛋白介导的细胞迁移。

肿瘤细胞通常表达高水平的唾液酸化的多糖，研究发现肿瘤细胞唾液酸化修饰的异常参与肿瘤的进展和侵袭。肿瘤细胞表面 Fas 受体的高度唾液酸化会使得结肠癌细胞对 Fas 介导的凋亡产生抵抗。此外，结肠癌中 EMT 的发生会引起唾液酸修饰酶的表达异常，进而上调唾液酸化的路易斯寡糖 x/a（sialyl Lewis x/a，sLe$^{x/a}$），而高表达的 sLe$^{x/a}$ 和肿瘤的侵袭以及患者的预后密切相关。胃癌细胞中 sLe$^{x/a}$ 表达水平升高，进而激活受体酪氨酸激酶 c – Met 及其下游的信号分子如 FAK（focal adhesion kinase，黏着斑激酶）和 Rac1 等，最终增强肿瘤细胞的侵袭能力，导致患者预后不良。

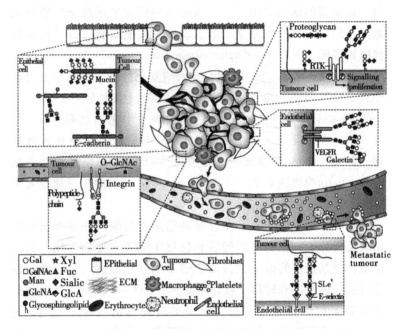

图 2 – 6　糖基化参与肿瘤的发生和发展

（引自 Nat Rev Cancer, 2015, 15: 540 – 555）

（三）蛋白糖基化修饰与肿瘤多药耐药

近年来，大量的研究表明糖蛋白糖基化修饰的改变对肿瘤耐药的产生起着至关重要的调节作用。据报道，用糖基化抑制剂衣霉素（tunicamycin）处理肿瘤耐药细胞可抑制耐药蛋白P-gp和BCRP（乳腺癌耐药蛋白）的N-糖基化修饰，进而逆转肿瘤细胞的耐药表型。我们实验室之前的研究发现，胃癌多药耐药关键分子P-gp在胃癌耐药细胞中糖基化修饰异常，且在糖基化位点Asn99处的糖基化修饰对其在胃癌多药耐药中功能的发挥十分重要。Lattova等的研究表明N-糖基化修饰的改变与乳腺癌细胞的化疗敏感性显著相关，且半乳糖或双天线型岩藻糖的增加可能和乳腺癌的耐药有关。此外，Nakano等发现在白血病细胞对埃博霉素（desoxyepothilone B）耐药的过程中，α2-6唾液酸化多糖的表达减少。Schultz等发现唾液酸转移酶ST6GAL1在顺铂耐药的肿瘤细胞中表达增高，且敲除ST6GAL1可使肿瘤细胞恢复对顺铂的敏感性，表明唾液酸化的异常参与肿瘤耐药的发生。Zhao等发现唾液酸转移酶ST6GAL1或ST8SIA2可以通过调节PI3K/AKT信号通路的活性来影响肝癌细胞的化疗敏感性。Cheng等的研究表明岩藻糖转移酶（fucosyltransferase，FUT）家族中的FUT4、FUT6和FUT8在肝癌多药耐药细胞中的表达显著升高，且能通过调节PI3K/AKT信号通路的活性和MRP1的表达来促进肝癌细胞多药耐药的产生。

（四）蛋白糖基化修饰研究现状

通过查阅文献，我们发现以往对蛋白糖基化修饰与肿瘤之间关系的研究大都着眼于蛋白的糖基化位点或蛋白的某一类型的糖基化修饰。但是，一个糖蛋白大都有多个糖基化位点，且一个糖基化位点也可能连接有多个糖链，这就使得蛋白的糖基化修饰十分复杂。完整的糖肽分析应该同时包括三方面的信息，即肽段序列、糖基化位点以及与特定位点相连的糖链结构。蛋白糖基化修饰的复杂性给糖蛋白糖基化修饰的全面解析带来了极大的挑战。

近年来，随着糖蛋白组学技术的不断发展，关于 N - 糖基化以及 O - 糖基化的位点特异性糖型解析的报道不断出现。例如，Shah 等通过对雄激素依赖以及非雄激素依赖前列腺癌细胞系的蛋白组以及糖蛋白组的综合解析，不仅确定了差异表达的糖蛋白，同时也鉴定出了糖蛋白糖基化占有率以及位点特异性糖型的差异。在此基础上，他们发现了岩藻糖修饰在两种细胞系之间的差别，并证明了岩藻糖的改变是由特定的岩藻糖转移酶和岩藻糖苷酶的表达变化引起的，为临床上前列腺癌的早期筛查以及肿瘤进展监测提供了可能的生物学标志物。

在之前的工作中，我们建立了大规模鉴定完整糖肽的糖蛋白组分析方法。通过这一方法我们对人胚胎肾细胞系 HEK 293T 的糖蛋白组进行了位点特异性糖基化修饰的细致解析，共鉴定到了2249 个完整糖肽，以及 453 个糖基化位点上的 1769 个位点特异性多糖。然而，迄今为止，对完整糖肽的大规模鉴定和定量仍存在着相当多的技术难点，尤其是对低丰度分泌型糖蛋白的分析而言。为此，我们构建了一套用于分析胃癌多药耐药相关分泌型糖蛋白糖基化修饰的方法，包括分泌蛋白的浓缩、完整糖肽的富集以及位点特异性糖型的鉴定。此外，我们还对分泌型糖蛋白的糖基化位点和位点特异性糖型进行了定量分析，重点关注了糖基化位点占有率以及与特定糖基化位点相连的多糖结构。我们认为对位点特异性糖基化修饰的全面解析可以帮助我们更好地阐明胃癌多药耐药发生的复杂分子机制，从而促进胃癌多药耐药相关分子标志物的发现，并提高化疗药物的疗效。

三、胃癌耐药相关分泌型糖蛋白的鉴定与筛选

胃癌多药耐药的产生严重影响着胃癌患者的预后，因此，有关胃癌多药耐药机制的研究对提高胃癌患者的生存以及生活质量具有非常重要的临床意义。本实验室多年来一直致力于对胃癌多药耐药机制的研究，为此我们以胃腺癌细胞系 SGC7901 为亲本细胞系，经过长春新碱以及阿霉素的长期诱导建立了胃癌多药耐药细胞系 SGC7901/VCR（vincristine，长春新碱）和 SGC7901/ADR（adriamycin，阿霉素）。之后，以这三株细胞系为胃癌多药耐药研究的细胞模型，我们通过基因组学以及蛋白组学等方法筛选出了大量与胃癌多药耐药相关的分子。然而，我们遗憾地发现这些分子都不能完全阐明胃癌多药耐药的发生机制。随着近年来人们对肿瘤微环境以及蛋白糖基化修饰认识的不断深入，我们认为在前期研究成果的基础上，推进这两个方面的研究对于解决胃癌多药耐药这一难题具有关键意义。

肿瘤细胞分泌蛋白对肿瘤多药耐药的发生具有十分重要的意义，且相当一部分肿瘤细胞分泌蛋白为糖基化蛋白，其在加工成熟分泌至胞外前都需经历糖基化修饰。鉴于糖基化修饰对糖蛋白的正确折叠、构象形成以及功能发挥的重要作用，全面解析胃癌细胞分泌型糖蛋白的位点特异性糖型在耐药过程中的变化将有助于我们阐明胃癌多药耐药的发生机制。

（一）胃癌细胞系分泌蛋白组数据集

总的来讲，我们从三株胃癌细胞系（SGC7901、SGC7901/ADR 和 SGC7901/VCR）中共鉴定到了 1033 个 N – 连接糖基化位

点（localization probability ＞ 0.75），这些糖基化位点对应于 436
个非冗余的 N - 糖基化蛋白。此外，我们共鉴定出了 2222 个高可
信的 N - 连接位点特异性糖型。之后，我们综合运用生物信息学
软件和 Uniprot 数据库来确定所鉴定到的蛋白是否为分泌型糖蛋
白，结果发现：272 个糖蛋白为分泌型糖蛋白，且可通过经典分
泌途径分泌至胞外，其中 134 个蛋白包含有 Uniprot 关键词"signal"或"secreted"，138 个蛋白经 SignalP 软件预测为分泌型糖蛋
白。此外，SecretomeP 软件分析发现 74 个蛋白可经非经典的分泌
途径分泌至胞外。总之，我们的结果表明，鉴定到总蛋白的 79%
可经多种不同的途径分泌至细胞培养液中，这一结果也从侧面证
明了我们的分泌蛋白糖基化分析方法的高效性。

　　为了进一步解析所鉴定到的分泌型糖蛋白，我们利用
PANTHER 软件对 346 个分泌型糖蛋白进行了分子功能和相关信号
通路的分析。结果发现，这些糖蛋白有着多种功能且参与了多个
信号通路，更重要的是这些分子功能和信号通路在肿瘤多药耐药
的发生中起着至关重要的作用。我们发现，这些分泌型糖蛋白所
具有的最主要的三种分子功能为催化活性（32.8%）、结合活性
（27.0%）以及受体活性（25.0%）。此外，这些分泌型糖蛋白参
与的和肿瘤多药耐药相关的主要分子通路为整联蛋白信号通路、
TGF - β 信号通路、cadherin 信号通路、血管新生、Wnt 信号通路
以及凋亡信号通路。

（二）胃癌多药耐药过程中 N - 糖基化位点占有率 的变化

　　与 SGC7901 相比，共有 240 个 N - 糖基化位点在 SGC 7901 -
ADR/VCR 中发生了显著的改变（124 个糖基化位点的占有率升
高，116 个糖基化位点的占有率降低）。此外，这些显著变化的糖

基化位点主要对应于 163 个糖基化蛋白，表达上调的糖基化位点对应于 84 个糖蛋白，表达下调的糖基化位点对应于 76 个糖蛋白，3 个糖蛋白同时包含上调的糖基化位点和下调的糖基化位点。进一步的生物信息学分析表明：上调的糖基化位点所对应的 87 个糖蛋白主要发挥结合活性（32.4%）、受体活性（25.4%）和催化活性（23.9%），而下调的糖基化位点所对应的 79 个糖蛋白所具有的分子功能主要为催化活性（33.3%）、受体活性（25.0%）和结合活性（25.0%）。

（三）胃癌多药耐药过程中位点特异性糖型的变化

我们发现只有核心岩藻糖以及复合型多糖在胃癌细胞产生获得性耐药以后发生了显著的变化，而其他几种重要的糖型并没有表现出明显的改变。此外，我们进一步确定了 SGC7901 和胃癌耐药细胞系之间明显差异的位点特异性糖型。共有 175 个位点特异性糖型在胃癌耐药细胞的分泌蛋白中显著上升，而 324 个位点特异性糖型在胃癌多药耐药细胞的分泌蛋白中显著下调。有意思的是，我们发现一些糖基化位点既连接有表达上调的糖型也连接有表达下降的糖型，这充分说明了糖基化修饰的高度复杂性。总的来讲，106 个糖蛋白中 151 个糖基化位点上的 499 个位点特异性糖型在胃癌多药耐药细胞和其亲本细胞中差异显著。对显著差异的位点特异性糖型所对应糖蛋白的深入分析发现大部分糖蛋白参与了 Integrin、P53、Wnt、Notch、TGF-beta 以及 Hedgehog 信号通路，且这些分子信号通路都在癌症的耐药产生中起着重要的作用

（四）胃癌多药耐药过程中显著差异的糖基化位点和位点特异性糖型的综合分析

我们发现显著差异的位点特异性糖型所对应的糖基化位点与

位点水平上显著变化的糖基化位点很少发生重合。此外，我们发现特定位点上所连接的差异表达的糖型不少于 2 个的糖蛋白共有 57 个，而这些糖蛋白中有 33 个已被报道和肿瘤的多药耐药相关，其中以 AXL、L1CAM、TIMP1 和 Clusterin 在肿瘤耐药中的研究最为广泛。这一结果也从侧面证明了蛋白糖基化修饰和肿瘤多药耐药密切相关。

（五） AXL 在胃癌多药耐药中作用的初步验证

我们发现 AXL mRNA 的表达在胃癌多药耐药细胞中显著上升；我们之前对三株细胞系的细胞蛋白进行了同位素标记定量质谱分析；通过分析数据，我们发现 AXL 蛋白在耐药细胞中的表达升高。此外，分泌型 AXL 在胃癌多药耐药细胞培养上清中的表达也有着明显的升高。更重要的是，基于 TCGA 数据库中的 295 例胃癌数据，我们发现胃癌组织中 AXL mRNA 的高表达预示着胃癌患者的预后不良。综上所述，我们首次证明了 AXL 在胃癌多药耐药过程中其糖基化修饰和蛋白表达都发生了显著的改变，提示分泌型 AXL 在胃癌多药耐药的产生中发挥着重要的作用。

总的来说，我们率先从蛋白质组学层面系统地研究了胃癌细胞分泌型糖蛋白的位点特异性糖基化修饰，证明了胃癌细胞分泌型糖蛋白的糖基化位点以及位点特异性糖型在细胞产生获得性多药耐药后发生了显著改变。此外，进一步的分析发现某些糖基化修饰异常的分泌型糖蛋白可能在胃癌多药耐药的进程中发挥着重要的作用，这一结果表明对特定糖蛋白糖基化修饰的调节可能成为逆转胃癌多药耐药的潜在治疗靶点。

（吴　键　聂勇战）

参考文献

[1] Sun Y. Tumor microenvironment and cancer therapy resistance. Cancer Lett, 2015,380(1):205 - 215.

[2] Quail DF, Joyce JA. Microenvironmental regulation of tumor progression and metastasis. Nat Med, 2013, 19: 1423 - 1437.

[3] Hui L, Chen Y. Tumor microenvironment: Sanctuary of the devil. Cancer Lett, 2015, 368: 7 - 13.

[4] Junttila MR, de Sauvage FJ. Influence of tumour micro - environment heterogeneity on therapeutic response. Nature, 2013, 501: 346 - 354.

[5] Song T, Dou C, Jia Y, et al. TIMP - 1 activated carcinoma - associated fibroblasts inhibit tumor apoptosis by activating SDF1/CXCR4 signaling in hepatocellular carcinoma. Oncotarget, 2015, 6: 12061 - 12079.

[6] Hirata E, Girotti MR, Viros A, et al. Intravital imaging reveals how BRAF inhibition generates drug - tolerant microenvironments with high integrin beta1/FAK signaling. Cancer Cell, 2015, 27: 574 - 588.

[7] Sun Y, Campisi J, Higano C, et al. Treatment - induced damage to the tumor microenvironment promotes prostate cancer therapy resistance through WNT16B. Nat Med, 2012, 18: 1359 - 1368.

[8] Ruffell B, Coussens LM. Macrophages and Therapeutic Resistance in Cancer. Cancer Cell, 2015, 27: 462 - 472.

[9] Weizman N, Krelin Y, Shabtay - Orbach A, et al. Macrophages mediate gemcitabine resistance of pancreatic adenocarcinoma by upregulating cytidine deaminase. Oncogene, 2014, 33: 3812 - 3819.

[10] Yang C, He L, He P, et al. Increased drug resistance in breast cancer by tumor - associated macrophages through IL - 10/STAT3/bcl - 2 signaling pathway. Med Oncol, 2015, 32: 352.

[11] Jahangiri A, Aghi MK, Carbonell WS. beta1 integrin: Critical path to antiangiogenic therapy resistance and beyond. Cancer Res, 2014, 74: 3 - 7.

[12] Chung AS, Wu X, Zhuang G, et al. An interleukin – 17 – mediated paracrine network promotes tumor resistance to anti – angiogenic therapy. Nat Med, 2013, 19: 1114 – 1123.

[13] Straussman R, Morikawa T, Shee K, et al. Tumour micro – environment elicits innate resistance to RAF inhibitors through HGF secretion. Nature, 2012, 487: 500 – 504.

[14] Obenauf AC, Zou Y, Ji AL, et al. Therapy – induced tumour secretomes promote resistance and tumour progression. Nature, 2015, 520: 368 – 372.

[15] Zhang FF, Zhu YF, Zhao QN, et al. Microvesicles mediate transfer of P – glycoprotein to paclitaxel – sensitive A2780 human ovarian cancer cells, conferring paclitaxel – resistance. Eur J Pharmacol, 2014, 738: 83 – 90.

[16] Choi DY, You S, Jung JH, et al. Extracellular vesicles shed from gefitinib – resistant nonsmall cell lung cancer regulate the tumor microenvironment. Proteomics, 2014, 14: 1845 – 1856.

[17] Xiu P, Dong X, Dong X, et al. Secretoryclusterin contributes to oxaliplatin resistance by activating Akt pathway in hepatocellular carcinoma. Cancer Sci, 2013, 104: 375 – 382.

[18] Huang H, Wang L, Li M, et al. Secretedclusterin (sCLU) regulates cell proliferation and chemosensitivity to cisplatin by modulating ERK1/2 signals in human osteosarcoma cells. World J Surg Oncol, 2014, 12: 255.

[19] Liu Z, Xu J, He J, et al. A critical role of autocrine sonic hedgehog signaling in human CD138 + myeloma cell survival and drug resistance. Blood, 2014, 124: 2061 – 2071.

[20] Yuan G, Regel I, Lian F, et al. WNT6 is a novel target gene of caveolin – 1 promoting chemoresistance to epirubicin in human gastric cancer cells. Oncogene, 2013, 32:375 – 387.

[21] Cho HJ, Kim IK, Park SM, et al. VEGF – C mediatesRhoGDI2 – induced gastric cancer cell metastasis and cisplatin resistance. Int J Cancer, 2014, 135: 1553 – 1563.

[22] Ohtsubo K, Marth JD. Glycosylation in cellular mechanisms of health and disease. Cell, 2006, 126: 855 – 867.

[23] Pinho SS, Reis CA. Glycosylation in cancer: mechanisms and clinical implications. Nat Rev Cancer, 2015, 15: 540 – 555.

[24] Pinho SS, Carvalho S, Marcos – Pinto R, et al. Gastric cancer: adding glycosylation to the equation. Trends Mol Med, 2013, 19: 664 – 676.

[25] Paredes J, Figueiredo J, Albergaria A, et al. Epithelial E – and P – cadherins: role and clinical significance in cancer. Biochim Biophys Acta, 2012, 1826: 297 – 311.

[26] Zhou F, Su J, Fu L, et al. Unglycosylation at Asn – 633 made extracellular domain of E – cadherin folded incorrectly and arrested in endoplasmic reticulum, then sequentially degraded by ERAD. Glycoconj J, 2008, 25: 727 – 740.

[27] Isaji T, Sato Y, Fukuda T, et al. N – glycosylation of the I – like domain of beta1 integrin is essential for beta1 integrin expression and biological function: identification of the minimal N – glycosylation requirement for alpha5beta1. J Biol Chem, 2009, 284: 12207 – 12216.

[28] Zhao Y, Nakagawa T, Itoh S, et al. N – acetylglucosaminyltransferase III antagonizes the effect of N – acetylglucosaminyltransferase V on alpha3beta1 integrin – mediated cell migration. J Biol Chem, 2006, 281: 32122 – 32130.

[29] Bull C, Stoel MA, den Brok MH, et al. Sialic acids sweeten a tumor's life. Cancer Res, 2014, 74: 3199 – 3204.

[30] Swindall AF, Bellis SL. Sialylation of the Fas death receptor by ST6Gal – I provides protection against Fas – mediated apoptosis in colon carcinoma cells. J Biol Chem, 2011, 286: 22982 – 22990.

[31] Sakuma K, Aoki M, Kannagi R. Transcription factors c – Myc and CDX2 mediate E – selectin ligand expression in colon cancer cells undergoing EGF/bFGF – induced epithelial – mesenchymal transition. Proc Natl Acad Sci USA, 2012, 109: 7776 – 7781.

[32] Gomes C, Osorio H, Pinto MT, et al. Expression of ST3GAL4 leads to SLe(x) expression and induces c – Met activation and an invasive phenotype in gastric carcinoma cells. PLoS One, 2013, 8: e66737.

[33] Wojtowicz K, Januchowski R, Nowicki M, et al. Inhibition of protein gly-cosylation reverses the MDR phenotype of cancer cell lines. Biomed Pharmacother, 2015, 74: 49 −56.

[34] Li K, Sun Z, Zheng J, et al. In − depth research of multidrug resistance related cell surfaceglycoproteome in gastric cancer. J Proteomics, 2013, 82: 130 −140.

[35] Lattova E, Bartusik D, Spicer V, et al. Alterations in glycopeptides associated with herceptin treatment of human breast carcinoma mcf − 7 and T − lymphoblastoid cells. Mol Cell Proteomics, 2011, 10: M111.007765.

[36] Lattova E, Tomanek B, Bartusik D, et al. N − glycomic changes in human breast carcinoma MCF − 7 and T − lymphoblastoid cells after treatment with herceptin and herceptin/Lipoplex. J Proteome Res, 2010, 9: 1533 −1540.

[37] Nakano M, Saldanha R, Gobel A, et al. Identification of glycan structure alterations on cell membrane proteins in desoxyepothilone B resistant leukemia cells. Mol Cell Proteomics, 2011, 10: M111.009001.

[38] Schultz MJ, Swindall AF, Wright JW, et al. ST6Gal − I sialyltransferase confers cisplatin resistance in ovarian tumor cells. J Ovarian Res, 2013, 6: 25.

[39] Zhao Y, Li Y, Ma H, et al. Modification ofsialylation mediates the invasive properties and chemosensitivity of human hepatocellular carcinoma. Mol Cell Proteomics, 2014, 13: 520 −536.

[40] Cheng L, Luo S, Jin C, et al. FUT family mediates the multidrug resistance of human hepatocellular carcinoma via the PI3K/Akt signaling pathway. Cell Death Dis, 2013, 4: e923.

[41] Shah P, Wang X, Yang W, et al. Integrated Proteomic and Glycoproteomic Analyses of Prostate Cancer Cells Reveal Glycoprotein Alteration in Protein Abundance and Glycosylation. Mol Cell Proteomics, 2015, 14: 2753 −2763.

[42] Hoffmann M, Marx K, Reichl U, et al. Site − specific O − Glycosylation Analysis of Human Blood Plasma Proteins. Mol Cell Proteomics, 2016,

15: 624 – 641.

[43] Sun S, Shah P, Eshghi ST, et al. Comprehensive analysis of protein glycosylation by solid – phase extraction of N – linked glycans and glycosite – containing peptides. Nat Biotechnol, 2016, 34: 84 – 88.

[44] Cheng K, Chen R, Seebun D, et al. Large – scale characterization of intact N – glycopeptides using an automated glycoproteomic method. J Proteomics, 2014, 110: 145 – 154.

第三章
Hsp90β1 介导 miR−23b−3p 调控胃癌多药耐药

一、胃癌研究的现状

在世界范围内，胃癌是常见的恶性肿瘤之一，根据世界卫生组织统计结果，2012 年全世界约有 951 000 例的新发病例，然而死于胃癌的病例竟多达 723 000 例。其中超过 70% 的病例发生在发展中国家，尤其是中国。我国一直都是胃癌的高发国家，其发病率占全球四成，死亡人数占 2/3，给社会和家庭带来了沉重的经济负担。在我国，由于胃癌早期诊断率低，胃癌患者明确诊断时大多已为中晚期，错过了手术治疗的最佳时间，此时单纯的手术治疗已无法根除病灶，新辅助化疗的出现就成为了进展期胃癌的主要治疗方法。治疗初期化疗药物往往会起到比较好的效果，但是随之而来的胃癌细胞的耐药却成为了治疗的一个巨大障碍。随着科技医疗的进步，新的药物不断涌现，虽然已有多种化疗药物和分子靶向药物应用于临床，但是胃癌患者的 5 年生存率仍不足 30%，最主要的原因就是胃癌多药耐药的产生。因此，明确胃癌多药耐药发生的机制，找到可有效逆转胃癌耐药的分子靶点，对提高胃癌患者的生存率至关重要。

二、肿瘤多药耐药及其相关分子机制

(一) 肿瘤多药耐药概述

化疗药物的出现，对肿瘤的治疗具有里程碑式的意义。然而，化疗药物的有效性却因固有性或获得性的多药耐药而大打折扣，甚至于无效。多药耐药（multidrug resistence，MDR）是指肿瘤细胞在对某种化疗药物发生耐药后，同时对药理和结构不同的其他尚未接触过的抗肿瘤药物也出现了交叉耐药的现象。在诸多肿瘤中，如胃癌、结肠癌、乳腺癌和卵巢癌，MDR 严重影响患者的预后与存活率。虽然医学研究的发展，为胃癌的临床治疗带来了新的化疗药物，胃癌的多药耐药现象成为阻碍胃癌患者预后的重要难题。因此深入研究肿瘤细胞 MDR 的机制、克服肿瘤的多药耐药性仍是世界性的热点问题，对改善患者预后、提高患者存活率至关重要。

(二) 肿瘤多药耐药相关机制研究

化学治疗是恶性肿瘤的首选治疗方法，然而多药耐药的产生却成为了化疗的一大障碍，能否预防或是逆转化疗耐药对肿瘤的治疗至关重要。耐药能够发生在多个层面，主要包括药物外排增加，改变药物靶点、DNA 损伤修复、细胞周期调控和逃避细胞凋亡。

1. 药物外排增加

药物外排的增加能够降低肿瘤细胞内化疗药物的有效浓度，是肿瘤细胞针对抗肿瘤制剂产生耐药的主要机制，这一过程主要依赖于一类转运性膜蛋白——ABC 转运蛋白。这类广泛存在于膜表面的超家族具有 ATP 依赖性，能够有效调控胞内药物复合体的吸收、分布和排泄。ABC 转运家族分为 ABCA ~ ABCG 7 个亚家族，其中至少有 12 个成员在药物转运的过程中起到重要作用，最常见的主要有 P - 糖蛋白（P - gp /ABCB1）、多药耐药相关蛋白（MRP1/ABCC1）和乳腺癌耐药蛋白（BCRP/ABCG2），P - gp 在肿瘤多药耐药方面的研究最为广泛。P - gp 分子量为 170 kDa，是由 7q21.1 染色体上的 ABCB1（MDR1）基因所编码，首次发现于中国仓鼠卵巢细胞的质膜。P - gp 能够通过 ATP 水解作用逆浓度梯度转运大量不同种类的分子，包括细胞生长抑制药物和内源性底物（类固醇激素、细胞因子）。研究证明，P - gp 高表达于乳腺癌、卵巢癌、膀胱癌、肺癌、口腔癌等多种肿瘤细胞中，并与上述肿瘤细胞化疗耐药的发生密切相关。

2. 药物靶点发生改变

化疗药物作用的靶点发生改变也能引起耐药的发生，这些改变既可以是质的变化，也可以是量的变化。药物活性的关键因素是 DNA 相关酶或细胞复制蛋白质。通过抗代谢物抑制关键酶（如 DNA 聚合酶、胸苷酸合成酶、核糖核苷酸合成酶）进而干扰核酸代谢，均可引起耐药的发生。例如胸苷酸合成酶水平的升高可诱发对氟尿嘧啶的耐药性。相反，下调 DNA 拓扑异构酶的水平可降低对蒽环类和喜树碱等重要抗瘤制剂的敏感性。耐紫杉醇也可与细胞内靶点的改变有关，包括微管蛋白水平的改变以及 α - 微管蛋白的乙酰化。通过 DNA 修复蛋白对药物（如顺铂）所致损伤的修复能力增强，也是导致细胞耐药的途径之一。核苷酸切除修复（NER）是铂类药物所致 DNA 损伤的主要途径，与 NER 相关的切除修复交叉互补基因 1 蛋白（ERCC1）已经临床前研究证明能够决定对顺铂的敏感性，其表达的增加会引起对顺铂的耐药性。

3. DNA 修复通路的改变

当化疗药物以 DNA 为靶点时，主要通过损伤肿瘤细胞的 DNA 以对抗肿瘤。而当基因组出现损伤时，DNA 反应性的通过损伤修复进行细胞的自我保护。肿瘤细胞同样会通过自身的修复或受损 DNA 的剔除来维持基因组的稳定性和完整性。DNA 损伤时，细胞通过细胞周期节点（G_1、S、G_2）通路进行反应，最终阻碍细胞周期蛋白依赖性激酶的活性进而导致细胞周期进程停滞。而这三个节点的作用在于除非 DNA 是完好的，否则 DNA 在受损状态下是无法进行复制的。可见，DNA 损伤修复能力的增强则与耐药有关。

4. 细胞凋亡的逃避

细胞凋亡是正常细胞程序性死亡的途径，确保了人体正常的新陈代谢。逃避凋亡是癌症的一个特征性的标志，是化疗耐药和放疗抵抗的一个重要组成部分，是肿瘤最具侵略性的一个特点。细胞凋亡的关键步骤与凋亡蛋白酶的激活有关，凋亡蛋白酶的激活主要存在以下两个途径：外源性的途径受到 TNF 受体家族的"死亡受体"的调控，包括 Fas（CD95/APO-1）、DR4（TNF-related apoptosis-inducing ligand receptor 1，TRAIL-R1）和 DR5（TRAIL-R2）；内源性途径则主要由 BCL2 调控。BCL2 是非常重要的一种抗凋亡基因，通过过表达和功能敲除的方法，BCL2 已被许多独立研究证明具有强大的对抗细胞凋亡的能力。研究报道 BCL2 参与胃癌、乳腺癌、肺癌、卵巢癌等多种肿瘤耐药的发生。p53 是另一个研究较多的凋亡相关基因，与BCL2 不同，p53 是一种抑癌基因，具有促进细胞凋亡的作用，主要是诱导 DNA 损伤细胞的凋亡。大多数恶性肿瘤已被证实存在 p53 的突变，导致药物所致凋亡受阻。p53 的突变与胃癌细胞的耐药亦密切相关，例如当联合使用 5-氟尿嘧啶和顺铂处理胃癌细胞时，与突变型 p53 的 MKN-28 细胞相比，野生型 p53 的MKN-45 细胞对上述两种药物更为敏感；另有研究发现胃癌耐药细胞中 Stat3 是处于过度激活的状态，当 Stat3 受到抑制后，其下游 p53 基因显著上调而 BCL2 和 c – Myc 基因的表达反而下降。因此，针对细胞凋亡相关分子的靶向性治疗，有望成为逆转肿瘤多药耐药的有效手段之一。

三、MicroRNA 与肿瘤耐药的研究

（一）MicroRNA 的概述

MicroRNA 是一类分子量非常小（21~25 个碱基）的内源性单链非蛋白编码 RNA，通过碱基互补配对原则与靶 mRNAs 的 3′UTR 区结合，在转录后水平调控基因的表达，可导致靶分子的 mRNA 降解或者翻译受抑制进而发挥相应的调控作用。

miRNAs 具有"一对多"的调控特点，单个 miRNA 可以多个靶基因 mRNA 进行调控，而单个 mRNA 又可受到多个 miRNAs 调控。MiRNAs 参与体内多种生物过程，包括细胞的生长、增殖、分化及凋亡等等。近年来，众多研究发现，miRNAs 的异常表达与肿瘤的发生、转移及多药耐药关系密切。miRNAs 对恶性肿瘤细胞的以下特性均具有调控作用：①细胞自我分泌生长因子（let – 7 家族）；②细胞对抗生长因子的抵抗性（miR – 17 – 92 cluster）；③凋亡逃逸（miR – 34a）；④细胞的无限增殖潜能（miR – 372/373 cluster）；⑤新生血管生成（miR –210）；⑥侵袭和转移（miR –10b）。相比于正常组织，肿瘤组织中 miRNAs 的表达或是上调或是下调，分别发挥着致瘤因子或肿瘤抑制因子的作用。因为 miRNAs 的表达有非常严格的组织特异性，故大量研究发现了不同肿瘤中 miRNAs 的表达模式，这使得 miRNAs 在临床应用中具有一定诊断和预后价值。

（二）MicroRNA 与肿瘤耐药

化疗耐药是肿瘤治疗过程中的一大关键问题。化疗耐药发生后，肿瘤细胞复发性的增殖并对具有更强的药物抵抗力，最终导致肿瘤复发或转移。MicroRNAs 是通过负性调控下游靶基因发挥作用的，其对肿瘤耐药表型的调控也是通过靶基因体现的。研究发现，不同肿瘤耐药表型主要与 microRNA 对细胞凋亡、细胞周期分布和药物外排转运体的异常调控实现的。表 3 – 1 是对部分耐药肿瘤及其相关 miRNAs 的归纳。

表 3 – 1　与肿瘤耐药相关 microRNAs

肿瘤类型	microRNAs	治疗药物	靶点
Breast cancer	miR – 328	MXR	ABCG
	miR – 221/222	Fulvestrant	p27，Kip1
	miR – 326	VP – 16/ADX	MRP – 1
	miR – 451	Irinotecan	ABCB1
	miR – 182	PARP1 inhibitor	BRCA1
Ovarian cancer	miR – 199a	CDD/PTX/ADR	ABCG2
	miR – 27a	PTX	MDR1/P – gp
Lung cancer	miR – 7	TKIs	EGFR
	miR – 103/203	TKIs	PKC /SRC
Colon cancer	miR – 19b/21	5 – FU	SFPQ，MYBL2
	miR – 215	MTX，TDX	DTL
	miR – 519c	MXR	ABCG2
Prostate cancer	miR – 34a	Camptothecin	CDK6，E2F3，E2F1
	miR – 148a	N. R.	MSK1
Gastric cancer	miR – 34a	ADX，CDD，GEM	Bcl2
	miR – 200b/c/429	CDD，VCR	Bcl – 2，Xiap
	miR – 508 – 5p	5 – FU，VCR	ABCB1，ZNRD1
	miR – 15b/16	ADR，VP – 16，CDD	Bcl – 2

　　胃癌多药耐药已被证明与多种 miRNAs 的异常表达有关，其中，miR - 15b/16 是首次发现的与胃癌 MDR 相关的 miRNAs。我室夏琳博士等发现，miR - 15b/16 通过负性调控抗凋亡基因 BCL2 的表达部分逆转胃癌多药耐药表型；我室尚玉龙博士等发现，miR - 508 - 5p 通过对基因 ABCB1 和 ZNRD1 的调控改善胃癌耐药细胞对药物的敏感性；miR - 21 和 miR - 106a 高表达于胃癌耐药细胞，分别抑制了抑癌基因 PTEN 和 RUNX3 的表达。表 3 - 2 是胃癌多药耐药中部分与 CPT、CDDP 和 CF 敏感性相关的 miRNAs。尽管 miRNAs 在包括胃癌耐药在内的多种肿瘤耐药中均发挥强大的调节功能，但目前临床上的收效甚微。因此，我们仍需更加深入的探索研究以 miRNAs 为靶点的治疗策略，以期进一步解决胃癌多药耐药这道难题。

表 3 - 2　与胃癌多药耐药相关的 microRNAs

---

5 - FU sensitivity

let - 7g

miR - 10b, - 22, - 30c, - 31, - 32

miR - 133b, - 143, - 144, - 145, - 181b, - 190, - 197, - 200c, - 204, - 210

miR - 335, - 501 - 5p, - 532, - 615, - 615 - 5p, - 766, - 877

miR - 1224 - 3p, - 1229, - 3131, - 3149, - 3162 - 3p, - 4763 - 3p

CPT sensitivity

let - 7g

miR - 7, - 31, - 98, - 126, - 196a, - 200, - 338

CDDP, CF sensitivity

let - 7g

miR - 1, - 16, - 21, - 34, - 181b, - 342, - 497

四、热休克蛋白与肿瘤的研究

(一) 热休克蛋白的研究概述

热休克蛋白 (heat shock proteins, HSPs), 是一类在进化上高度保守的多肽蛋白质, 是 Ritossa 在 1962 年研究亚致死性热应力对随后的致死性损伤具有保护作用时首次发现的。热休克蛋白几乎存在于所有的生物体中, 当细胞受到各种不同的生理或环境刺激条件时, 包括高温、氧自由基、氨基酸类似物、重金属、乙醇等等, 其表达升高, 此外临床缺血/再灌注损伤和各种炎症性疾病的情况也会引起热休克反应。分子伴侣功能是热休克蛋白最重要的功能, 它们在体内参与维持蛋白多肽的正确组装、平衡蛋白的合成与降解、参与蛋白的准确定位等等重要的生理过程。HSPs 对细胞还具有保护功能, 当细胞受到各种刺激时, 胞内的 HSPs 迅速升高, 保护细胞免受内源性应激的损害, 并增强细胞的修复能力。在人体内, 某一种 HSP 或是 HSP 伴侣复合体与新合成的、构想不稳定的蛋白多肽结合, 通过以下方式对其进行调控: ①帮助蛋白质避免其发生聚合; ②协助蛋白质的细胞内转运, 特别是跨膜转运; ③维持蛋白质的稳定性并辅助其功能的发挥; ④当缺乏有效刺激时, 可通过泛素化-蛋白酶体途径使蛋白发生降解, 以维持胞内蛋白表达水平的相对稳定。很多疾病的发生与蛋白质缺陷有关, 如帕金森神经退行性疾病、阿尔茨海默病、亨廷顿病和朊病毒相关疾病等, 故 HSPs 与人类的许多疾病的发生、发展也有着密切的关系。近年来多项研究发现, HSPs 在多种不同类型的肿瘤中呈高表达状态。HSPs 是个多基因家族, 人们常常根据分子量的大小将 HSPs 分为以下几类：大分子 HSPs（≥100 kDa）、HSP90（81 ~ 99 kDa）、HSP70（65 ~ 80 kDa）、HSP60（55 ~ 64 kDa）、HSP40（35 ~ 54 kDa）以及小分子 HSPs（≤34 kDa）。

（二）热休克蛋白 90 与肿瘤

Hsp90 是到目前为止研究最广泛的肿瘤治疗靶点。Hsp90 是一类含量丰富、高度保守的分子伴侣。正常情况下，Hsp90 占人体蛋白总量的 1% ~ 2%，当受到刺激诱发时，其可增至蛋白总量的 4% ~ 6%。Hsp90 对细胞内超过 200 种蛋白质具有调控作用，其中它对许多与肿瘤发生、发展相关的作用蛋白的稳定和功能至关重要，这些作用蛋白是多数致癌信号通路中的关键蛋白，如络氨酸激酶受体（EGFR、HER2、c - KIT、MEK、VEGFR、FLT3、IGFR1）、信号转导蛋白（BCR - ABL、ALK、BRAF、AKT）、转录因子（雄激素和雌激素受体、HIF1α、P53）、细胞周期调控蛋白（CDK4、RB、cyclin D）、抗凋亡蛋白（BCL2、survivin）以及端粒酶（hTERT、MMP2、MIF），见图 3 - 1。Hsp90 参与了肿瘤细胞的增殖、侵袭、转移以及血管生成等一系列重要过程。①Hsp90 可促进肿瘤细胞恶性转化：肿瘤细胞具有无限增值的能力，但这些都离不开许多转录因子、蛋白激酶等蛋白的帮助，Hsp90 具有稳定这些蛋白的功能并可使信号蛋白维持在待激活的状态；此外，Hsp90 还能稳定并结合突变蛋白，使肿瘤细胞持续发生恶性转化。②Hsp90 可抑制细胞的衰老：端粒酶稳定性的维持离不开 Hsp90，在正常细胞中，随着染色体的分裂，端粒也会逐渐缩短，直至细胞无法继续分裂，而在肿瘤细胞中，因为端粒酶的表达通常是上调的，端粒酶修复延长了端粒，细胞获得了不断分裂的能力。③Hsp90 促进肿瘤新生血管生成：转录因子 HIF1α 参与调控新生血管的生成，其下

游通路的血管内皮生长因子和一氧化氮合成酶也都与血管内皮
细胞的增殖和迁移有关，而这些分子的稳定性和激活都离不开
Hsp90。这说明 Hsp90 对新生血管的生成非常重要。④Hsp90 促
进肿瘤细胞的侵袭和转移：已有研究证明，抑制 Hsp90 的表达
可抑制肝细胞生长因子 – met – 尿激酶型纤溶酶原激活物 – 血纤
维蛋白溶酶通路，最终降低肿瘤细胞浸润和迁移的能力；由上
皮生长因子所致的甲状腺癌细胞的侵袭能力，也可通过对 Hsp90
的抑制而得到改善。

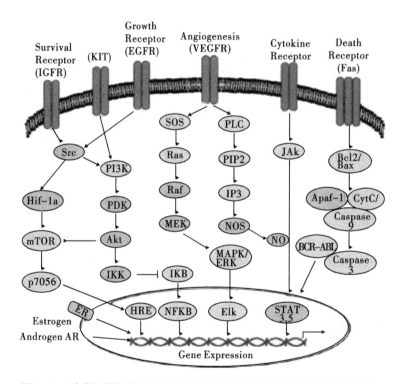

图 3 – 1 肿瘤细胞存活和抗凋亡相关的 HSP90 下游作用蛋白及其信号通路

（引自 Cancer Treat Rev，2013，39：375 – 387）

（三）Hsp90β1 与肿瘤的研究现状

Hsp90 家族由 5 个亚家族 17 种基因成员组成，其中的 6 种基因成员已被认定是在人体发挥作用的，包括 Hsp90α 亚家族的成员 Hsp90AA1、Hsp90AA2、Hsp90N、Hsp90AB1 和 Hsp90β 亚家族的 Hsp90β1 和 TRAP1。Hsp90β 是 Hsp90 调控细胞结构的维持、细胞分化和细胞自我保护等正常细胞功能的主要形式。Hsp90β1 作为 Hsp90β 亚家族最主要的成员，具有应激后帮助细胞存活及变性蛋白复性的功能。有研究证明，Hsp90β1 可通过协助细胞逃逸凋亡和保存各种原癌基因功能的方式促进乳腺癌生长。Zongguo Yang 等研究表明，肝癌组织中 Hsp90β1 表达上调，且与较差的存活率相关。另有研究证明，骨肉瘤中 Hsp90β1 起到致癌基因的作用，并且受到 miR - 223 的直接调控。可见，Hsp90β1 与肿瘤也有着密切的关系。此外，有研究报道在肿瘤耐药细胞中下调 Hsp90 的表达可以明显逆转 ABCB1 依赖的耐药表型。刘等通过免疫组化和原位杂交的方法发现，Hsp90β 在胃癌耐药细胞系 SGC7901/VCR 中表达高于其亲本细胞。

目前，关于 Hsp90β1 与包括胃癌在内的肿瘤耐药的相关研究报道为数不多，刘的研究也只是说明了 Hsp90β 高表达于胃癌耐药细胞中。Hsp90β1 是通过何种机制调控胃癌耐药尚不清楚，所以我们认为关于 Hsp90β1 与胃癌多药耐药的关系，以及与之相关的 Hsp90β1 的上下游调节通路尚需进一步研究说明。

五、Hsp90β1在介导miR-23b-3p调控胃癌多药耐药中的作用

　　在肿瘤细胞中，HSPs保护细胞免受凋亡的能力可促进肿瘤的发生、发展。Hsp90β1作为一种新的亚型分子，是Hsp90β最主要的成员，我们前期研究发现，其在胃癌耐药细胞系中的表达常常是上调的，因此我们推测Hsp90β1与胃癌的多药耐药有关。此外，本课题组前期通过进行胃癌多药耐药表型相关miR-NAs的高通量功能获得性筛选，发现了多个能明显逆转胃癌多药耐药的miRNAs，其中miR-23b-3p的作用最为明显。有意思的是，在通过生物信息学软件对Hsp90β1 3'-UTR区进行反向预测的结果中，我们发现了多个miRNA的结合位点，其中就有miR-23b-3p。于是我们再次利用生物信息学软件分析预测miR-23b-3p的下游靶基因，并筛选到了Hsp90β1和另外两个耐药经典分子ABCB1和BCL2。由此，我们可以推测胃癌耐药重要分子Hsp90β1可能介导miR-23b-3p对胃癌多药耐药的负性调控。基于这个问题，我们开展了本实验研究，深入探讨miR-23b-3p-Hsp90β1轴在胃癌多药耐药的生物学功能和分子机制。并结合生物信息学软件分析预测靶基因的结果，将经典耐药相关分子ABCB1和BCL2一并纳入研究。本实验一方面通过耐药相关细胞功能学实验（MTT药敏实验、流式细胞凋亡实验及ADR药物蓄积实验）验证了Hsp90β1的促耐药作用和miR-23b-3p的抑制耐药作用；另一方面，通过qRT-PCR、Western blot和荧光素酶报告基因实验明确了Hsp90β1对其下游作用蛋白ABCB1和BCL2的调控以及miR-23b-3p负性调控基因Hsp90β1、ABCB1和BCL2的作用。

综上所述，Hsp90β1 通过对耐药分子 ABCB1 和 BCL2 的调控进而介导了 miR – 23b – 3p 的胃癌耐药调控作用，而 miR – 23b – 3p 亦可通过直接作用于 ABCB1 和 BCL2 而调控胃癌多药耐药。

（郭　阳）

参考文献

［1］　Torre LA, Bray F, Siegel RL, et al. Global cancer statistics, 2012. CA Cancer J Clin, 2015, 65: 87 – 108.

［2］　Zhao X, Li Y, Hu J. Down – regulation of miR – 27a might inhibit proliferation and drug resistance of gastric cancer cells. J Exp Clin Cancer Res, 2011, 30: 2351 – 2354.

［3］　Li J, Zhang Y, Zhao J, et al. Overexpression of miR – 22 reverses paclitaxel – induced chemoresistance through activation of PTEN signaling in p53 – mutated colon cancer cells. Mol Cell Biochem, 2011, 357: 31 – 38.

［4］　Kastl L, Brown I, Schofield AC. miRNA – 34a is associated with docetaxel resistance in human breast cancer cells. Breast Cancer Res Treat, 2012, 131: 445 – 454.

［5］　Ye G, Fu G, Cui S, et al. MicroRNA 376c enhances ovarian cancer cell survival by targeting activin receptor – like kinase 7: implications for chemoresistance. J Cell Sci, 2011, 124: 359 – 368.

［6］　Sadegh M, Manfred S. Development of gastric cancer and its prevention. Arch Iran Med, 2014, 17: 514 – 520.

［7］　Wong R, Cunningham D. Optimising treatment regimens for the management of advanced gastric cancer. Ann Oncol, 2009, 20: 605 – 608.

［8］　Marin JJ, Romero MR, Blazquez AG, et al. Importance and limitations of chemotherapy among the available treatments for gastrointestinal tumours. Anticancer Agents Med Chem, 2009, 9: 162 – 184.

[9] Hummel R, Hussey DJ. MicroRNAs: predictors and modifiers of chemo - and radiotherapy in different tumour types. Eur J Cancer, 2010, 46: 298 - 311.

[10] Dean M, Hamon Y, Chimini G. The human ATP - binding cassette (ABC) transporter superfamily. Genome Res, 2001, 11: 1007 - 1017.

[11] Gillet JP, Efferth T, Remacle J. Chemotherapy - induced resistance by ATP - binding cassette transporter genes. Biochimica Et Biophysica Acta, 2007, 1775: 237 - 262.

[12] Zhang F, Zhang H, Wang Z, et al. P - glycoprotein associates with Anxa2 and promotes invasion in multidrug resistant breast cancer cells. Biochem Pharmacol, 2014, 87: 292 - 302.

[13] Zhu Y, Liu C, Nadiminty N, et al. Inhibition of ABCB1 expression overcomes acquired docetaxel resistance in prostate cancer. Mol Cancer Ther, 2013, 12: 1829 - 1836.

[14] Wang J, Zhang J, Zhang L, et al. Expression of P - gp, MRP, LRP, GST - π andTopoIIα and intrinsic resistance in human lung cancer cell lines. Oncol Rep, 2011, 26: 1081 - 1089.

[15] Zhu H, Liu Z, Tang L, et al. Reversal of P - gp and MRP1 - mediated multidrug resistance by H6, agypenoside aglycon from Gynostemma pentaphyllum , in vincristine - resistant human oral cancer (KB/VCR) cells. Eur J Pharmacol, 2012, 696: 43 - 53.

[16] Casorelli I, Bossa C, Bignami M. DNA damage and repair in human cancer: molecular mechanisms and contribution to therapy - related leukemias. Int J Environ Res Public Health, 2012, 9: 2636 - 2657.

[17] Xia L, Zhang D, Du R, et al. miR - 15b and miR - 16 modulate multidrug resistance by targeting BCL2 in human gastric cancer cells. Int J Cancer, 2008, 123: 372 - 379.

[18] Huang S, Chen M, Shen Y, et al. Inhibition of activated Stat3 reverses drug resistance to chemotherapeutic agents in gastric cancer cells. Cancer Lett, 2012, 315: 198 - 205.

[19] Song JH, Meltzer SJ. MicroRNAs in pathogenesis, diagnosis, and treatment of gastroesophageal cancers. Gastroenterology, 2012, 143:35 - 47.

[20] Isabelle B, Neus R, Xin H, et al. Notch – mediated repression of bantam miRNA contributes to boundary formation in the Drosophila wing. Development, 2011, 138: 3781 – 3789.

[21] Yan G, Zhang L, Fang T, et al. MicroRNA – 145 suppresses mouse granulosa cell proliferation by targeting activin receptor IB. FEBS Lett, 2012, 586: 3263 – 3270.

[22] Garofalo M, Romano G, Leva GD, et al. EGFR and MET receptor tyrosine kinase – altered microRNA expression induces tumorigenesis and gefitinib resistance in lung cancers. Nat Med, 2011, 18: 74 – 82.

[23] Hansjuerg A, Cristian T, Hongping C, et al. Dysregulation of miR – 31 and miR – 21 induced by zinc deficiency promotes esophageal cancer. Carcinogenesis, 2012, 33: 1736 – 1744.

[24] Leva GD, Garofalo M, Croce CM. MicroRNAs in Cancer. Ann Rev Pathol, 2013, 9: 202 – 216.

[25] Pan YZ, Morris ME, Yu AM. MicroRNA – 328 negatively regulates the expression of breast cancer resistance protein (BCRP/ABCG2) in human cancer cells. Mol Pharmacol, 2009, 75: 1374 – 1379.

[26] Rao X, Leva GD, Li M, et al. MicroRNA – 221/222 confers breast cancer fulvestrant resistance by regulating multiple signaling pathways. Oncogene, 2011, 30: 1082 – 1097.

[27] Liang Z, Hui W, Xia J, et al. Involvement of miR – 326 in chemotherapy resistance of breast cancer through modulating expression of multidrug resistance – associated protein 1. Biochem Pharmacol, 2010, 79: 817 – 824.

[28] Rai K, Takigawa N, Ito S, et al. Liposomal Delivery of MicroRNA – 7 – Expressing Plasmid Overcomes Epidermal Growth Factor Receptor Tyrosine Kinase Inhibitor – Resistance in Lung Cancer Cells. Mol Cancer Ther, 2011, 10: 1720 – 1727.

[29] Kurokawa K, Tanahashi T, Iima T, et al. Role of miR – 19b and its target mRNAs in 5 – fluorouracil resistance in colon cancer cells. J Gastroenterol, 2012, 47: 883 – 895.

[30] Cheng W, Liu T, Wan X, et al. MicroRNA – 199a targets CD44 to sup-

press the tumorigenicity and multidrug resistance of ovarian cancer – initiating cells. FEBS J, 2012, 279: 2047 – 2059.

[31] Garofalo M, Romano G, Leva GD, et al. EGFR and MET receptor tyrosine kinase – altered microRNA expression induces tumorigenesis and gefitinib resistance in lung cancers. Nat Med, 2011, 18: 74 – 82.

[32] Keitaro K, Riyako O, Yasunori F, et al. A role for SIRT1 in cell growth and chemoresistance in prostate cancer PC3 and DU145 cells. Biochem Biophys Res Commun, 2008, 373: 423 – 428.

[33] Li Z, Hu S, Wang J, et al. MiR – 27a modulates MDR1/P – glycoprotein expression by targeting HIPK2 in human ovarian cancer cells. Gynecol Oncol, 2010, 119: 125 – 130.

[34] Bitarte N, Bandres E, Boni V, et al. MicroRNA – 451 is involved in the self – renewal, tumorigenicity, and chemoresistance of colorectal cancer stem cells. Stem Cells, 2011, 29: 1661 – 1671.

[35] Moskwa P, Buffa FM, Pan Y, et al. miR – 182 – mediated downregulation of BRCA1 impacts DNA repair and sensitivity to PARP inhibitors. Mol Cell, 2011, 41: 210 – 220.

[36] Song B, Wang Y, Titmus MA, et al. Molecular mechanism of chemoresistance by miR – 215 in osteosarcoma and colon cancer cells. Mol Cancer, 2010, 9: 96.

[37] Ji Q, Hao X, Meng Y, et al. Restoration of tumor suppressor miR – 34 inhibits human p53 – mutant gastric cancertumorspheres. BMC Cancer, 2008, 8: 1 – 12.

[38] Zhu W, Xu H, Zhu DX, et al. miR – 200bc/429 cluster modulates multidrug resistance of human cancer cell lines by targeting BCL2 and XIAP. Cancer Chemother Pharmacol, 2012, 69: 723 – 731.

[39] Shang Y, Zhang Z, Liu Z, et al. miR – 508 – 5p regulates multidrug resistance of gastric cancer by targeting ABCB1 and ZNRD1. Oncogene, 2014, 33: 3267 – 3276.

[40] Yasunori F, Keitaro K, Riyako O, et al. MiR – 148a attenuates paclitaxel resistance of hormone – refractory, drug – resistant prostate cancer PC3 cells

by regulating MSK1 expression. J Biol Chem, 2010, 285: 19076 – 19084.

[41] Yang SM, Huang C, Li XF, et al. miR – 21 confers cisplatin resistance in gastric cancer cells by regulating PTEN. Toxicology, 2013, 306: 162 – 168.

[42] Zhang Y, Lu Q, Cai X. MicroRNA – 106a induces multidrug resistance in gastric cancer by targeting RUNX3. FEBS Lett, 2013, 587: 3069 – 3075.

[43] Ishiguro H, Kimura M,Takeyama H. Role of microRNAs in gastric cancer. World J Gastroenterol, 2014, 20: 5694 – 5699.

[44] Taipale M, Jarosz DS. HSP90 at the hub of protein homeostasis: emerging mechanistic insights. Nat Rev Mol Cell Biol, 2010, 11: 515 – 528.

[45] Normant E, Paez G, West KA, et al. The Hsp90 inhibitor IPI – 504 rapidly lowers EML4 – ALK levels and induces tumor regression in ALK – driven NSCLC models. Oncogene, 2011, 30: 2581 – 2586.

[46] Len N, Paul W. Hsp90 molecular chaperone inhibitors: are we there yet. Clin Cancer Res, 2012, 18: 64 – 76.

[47] Mahalingam D, Swords R, Carew JS, et al. Targeting HSP90 for cancer therapy. Brit J Cancer, 2009, 100: 1523 – 1529.

[48] Shimamura T, Li D, Ji H, et al. Hsp90 inhibition suppresses mutant EGFR – T790M signaling and overcomes kinase inhibitor resistance. Cancer Res, 2008, 68: 5827 – 5838.

[49] Park Y, Kubo A,Komiya T, et al. Low – penetrant RB allele in small – cell cancer shows geldanamycin instability and discordant expression with mutant ras. Cell Cycle, 2008, 7: 2384 – 2391.

[50] Hong DS,Udai B, Bahareh T, et al. Targeting the molecular chaperone heat shock protein 90 (HSP90): lessons learned and future directions. Cancer Treat Rev, 2013, 39: 375 – 387.

[51] Powers MV, Paul W. Inhibitors of the heat shock response: biology and pharmacology. FEBS Lett, 2007, 581: 3758 – 3769.

[52] Yang Z, Zhuang L,Szatmary P, et al. Upregulation of heat shock proteins (HSPA12A, HSP90B1, HSPA4, HSPA5 and HSPA6) in tumour tissues is associated with poor outcomes from HBV – related early – stage hepatocellular carcinoma. Int J Med Sci, 2015, 12: 256 – 263.

[53] Li G, Cai M, Fu D, et al. Heat shock protein 90B1 plays an oncogenic role and is a target ofmicroRNA‑223 in human osteosarcoma. Cell Physiol Biochem, 2012, 30: 1481‑1490.

[54] Zhang H, Neely L, Lundgren K, et al. BIIB021, a synthetic Hsp90 inhibitor, has broad application against tumors with acquired multidrug resistance. Int J Cancer, 2010, 126: 1226‑1234.

[55] Len N, Paul W. Hsp90 molecular chaperone inhibitors: are we there yet? Clin Cancer Res, 2012, 18: 64‑76.

[56] Workman P, Powers MV. Chaperoning cell death: a critical dual role forHsp90 in small‑cell lung cancer. Nat Chem Biol, 2007, 3: 455‑457.

第四章

FNDC3B 介导 microRNA let-7f-5p
抑制胃癌转移

一、胃癌转移的主要分子生物学机制

胃癌是世界范围内最常见的恶性肿瘤之一，最新的统计结果表明，在我国胃癌的发病率及死亡率居所有肿瘤的第二位，仅次于肺癌。随着我国医疗水平的提高和人们健康意识不断增强，我国胃癌的发病率有所下降，但是其死亡率依然居高不下，胃癌患者的五年生存率更是只有 20% 左右。究其原因，胃癌患者高死亡率主要是由于胃癌发生转移所导致的。胃癌可在其发生、发展的各个阶段发生转移，当胃癌发生肝转移、腹膜转移或远处淋巴结转移时，手术、放疗、化疗等各种治疗手段均无法彻底清除胃癌及其转移灶，这是导致胃癌患者死亡的主要原因。

肿瘤转移是一个涉及多步骤、多阶段的生物学过程，可以分为以下几个步骤：由原发肿瘤细胞从相邻细胞中穿出开始，之后经过转移的肿瘤细胞通过血管内皮进入血液循环（intravasate）、肿瘤细胞随血液循环系统转移且在其中存活、移出血管（extravasate），最终在新的微环境中定植并增殖，形成在临床上可以检测到的转移灶。

参与肿瘤转移的相关基因及其蛋白产物大致可以分为以下几类。①蛋白溶解酶：包括基质金属蛋白酶（matrix metallopro-

teinase）、丝氨酸蛋白溶酶、半胱氨酸蛋白酶（cysteine protea-
ses），肿瘤细胞可以通过分泌这些蛋白溶解酶来破坏基底膜表面
的细胞基质或者基底膜，达到侵入周围组织和（或）穿越基底
膜的目的。②细胞黏附分子：主要有整合素（integrins）、钙黏
着蛋白（cadherins）、免疫球蛋白超家族和选择素家族（selec-
tins），这些蛋白大多分布在细胞膜上，可以介导细胞与细胞之
间和（或）细胞与细胞基质受体之间的相互作用，导致肿瘤细
胞之间和（或）肿瘤细胞与细胞基底膜之间的黏附能力减弱，
从而可以使肿瘤细胞从原发肿瘤灶脱落。③细胞因子：主要有
血管内皮生长因子（vascular endothelial growth factor，VEGF）、
肿瘤坏死因子-α（tumor necrosis factor-α，TNF-α）、胰岛素
样生长因子（insulin-like growth factor，IGF）等，这些生长因
子的作用主要是通过诱导新生血管形成、参与肿瘤细胞免疫逃
逸等途径促进肿瘤微转移灶的生长。

　　由此可见，肿瘤转移的发生、发展是一个涉及多基因、多
信号通路改变所导致的共同结果，这些与转移相关的因素相互
影响形成一个复杂的调控网络，在肿瘤转移的不同阶段均发挥
着重要的作用。

二、MicroRNA 在肿瘤发生、发展中发挥的重要作用

　　MicroRNAs（miRNAs）是一类含有 22～24 个核苷酸的内源
性单链 RNA，miRNA 主要是通过调节转录和（或）调节翻译蛋
白编码基因过程从而发挥其生物学功能。microRNA 首先在细胞
核内由基因组转录为初级 miRNA（pri-miRNA），之后在细胞
核内经过剪切形成 miRNA 的前体（pre-miRNA），pre-miRNA
转运到细胞质中经过 Drosha、Dicer 的加工生成成熟的 miRNA，

miRNA 发挥生物学功能主要是通过与募集 RISC 复合物后与 mRNA的 3′非编码区（3′-UTR）结合，从而导致靶基因 mRNA 的降解或者是导致翻译抑制来影响靶基因的表达，大多数 miRNA通过负性调节靶基因发挥其功能，但是研究发现有些 miRNA 也可以通过与 mRNA 的 5′非编码区（5′-UTR）结合使 mRNA 降解或抑制转录，有些 miRNA 甚至可以促进 mRNA 的 翻译。

（一） miRNA 在肿瘤中失调的相关分子机制

过去十年的研究发现 miRNA 在人恶性肿瘤中表达失调，主要的机制包括染色质异常、转录调控的变化、表观遗传的变化及 miRNA 生物合成过程中的缺陷。

1. miRNA 基因的扩增或者缺失

在恶性肿瘤中异常的 miRNA 表达归因于 miRNA 基因拷贝数和基因座位的改变。最早发现 miRNA 基因座位的变化是 miR-15a/16-1 基因簇在基因组 13q14 的缺失，这个现象常常在慢性 B 细胞白血病的患者中发现；相反的，在 B 细胞淋巴瘤的患者中 miR-17-92 基因簇扩增，从而导致 B 细胞淋巴瘤的恶性度增加；在 227 个人类卵巢癌、乳腺癌及黑素瘤样品中，运用基于阵列的高分辨率的基因组比较 miRNA 基因位点发现其基因组的高频改变。进一步对全基因组研究显示许多 miRNA 基因位于癌症相关的基因组区域。这些区域可以由于发生杂合性缺失从而导致肿瘤抑制基因微小区域的改变，这些区域可能包含癌基因或者脆弱的断裂位点。总之，这些发现表明 mRNA 在恶性肿瘤中的异常表达可能是由于 miRNA 特定基因组的扩增或者缺失引起的从而导致恶性肿瘤的发生。

2. miRNA 的转录调控作用

miRNA 的表达受到不同转录因子的调控，所以在肿瘤中

miRNA 的异常表达可能是由于一些关键转录因子（如 c - Myc 和 p53）的调控异常导致的。

O'Donnell 等人发现 c - Myc 常常在恶性肿瘤中高表达，其可调节肿瘤细胞的增殖和凋亡。c - Myc 可以通过激活 miR - 17 - 92 的 microRNA 簇从而发挥其促癌的功能，与其致癌作用一致，c - Myc 也抑制有肿瘤转录活性的 miRNA，如 miR - 15a、miR - 26、miR - 29、miR - 30 和 let - 7 家族；本实验室的赵晓迪博士，通过对促进胃癌转移的转录因子 SRF（serum response factor，血清应答因子）的研究，发现 SRF 可以直接结合 miR - 199a - 5p 的 3′ - UTR 区发挥其促进胃癌转移的作用；p53 - miR - 34 轴是转录因子调节 miRNA 表达从而介导其抑制肿瘤作用的另一个例子，p53 是肿瘤抑制基因由 TP53 基因编码，Oren 实验室发现 p53 可以通过直接结合启动子下调 miR - 34a 的表达从而促进癌细胞的凋亡。除了 c - Myc 和 p53 这两个研究最多的转录因子之外，还有诸多转录因子如 C/EBP/NFI - A 均可通过与 miRNA 结合调节肿瘤的发生、发展。Fazi 等人发现 miR - 223 和转录因子 NFI - A 和 C /EBPα 形成一个调控环路控制人粒细胞分化。这两个转录因子竞争结合 miR - 223 的启动子，NFI - A 使 miR - 223 保持在较低水平，而视黄酸诱导的 C /EBPα 取代 NFI - A 上调 miR - 223 的表达。因此，miRNA 的表达受到多种因素的调整，以维持正常的转录，其失调导致肿瘤发生。

3. miRNA 生成机制障碍

miRNA 的生成需要某些酶及调控蛋白的调节，如 Drosha、Dicer、DGCR8 等，当 miRNA 合成过程中的任意组成条件发生改变就会引起 miRNA 表达的变化从而引起肿瘤的发生、发展。Drosha 和 Dicer 是在 miRNA 成熟过程中的两个关键酶，研究表明，这两个催化酶在肿瘤中有不同程度的失调，有研究表明，在卵巢癌中高表达的 Drosha 和 Dicer 伴随着高生存率，相反的，低表达 Dicer 与患者的生存率的降低明显相关；Walz 等人发现在 15% Wilm's 肉瘤中 DGCR8 和 Drosha 出现单个碱基的缺失突变，导致成熟 let-7a 和 miR-200 家族表达的减少，可能与 Wilm's 肉瘤的发生有关。

4. 表观遗传变化的失调

表观遗传学改变是癌症公认的特征，包括全基因组 DNA 甲基化、肿瘤抑制基因的 DNA 异常甲基化及组蛋白修饰模式异常。miRNA 类似于蛋白质编码基因，也容易受到表观遗传的影响。例如，Fazi 等人发现 miR-223 表达被一个最常见的白血病相关融合蛋白 AML1／ETO 通过 CpG 甲基化表观遗传学沉默。Saito 等人发现当使用 DNA 甲基化和组蛋白乙酰化抑制剂同时治疗后在人 313 个 miRNA 中有 17 个在 T24 膀胱癌细胞中上调三倍。在这些 miRNA 中，miR-127，嵌入 CpG 岛而且在癌细胞中缺乏表达，当治疗后伴随原癌基因 BCL6 的下调 miR-223 的表达显著升高。这些结果表明，DNA 去甲基化和组蛋白脱乙酰抑制剂可以激活的 miRNA 的表达从而作为肿瘤抑制剂。类似的，Lujambio 等人发现 miR-148a 和 miR-34b／c 簇可在癌细胞中被特异性超甲基化沉默。此外，在肿瘤细胞中这些 miRNA 可抑制其肿瘤细胞的移动、抑制肿瘤的生长和抑制转移的形成。同时 miR-9-1、miR-124a 和 miR-145-5p 的表达降低会导致乳腺癌，肺癌和结肠癌的 DNA 甲基化。上述证据突出肿瘤发生过程中 miRNA 表达表观遗传在肿瘤中的调控作用，提示 miRNA 基因的异常 DNA 甲基化和组蛋白乙酰化可以作为癌症诊断和预后的生物标志物。

（二）在肿瘤中 miRNA 表达改变的意义

Hanahan 和 Weinberg 等人发现在肿瘤的发生、发展过程中肿瘤获得六个生物功能标志，包括获得持续性生长信号、逃避生长抑制、抑制细胞死亡、获得持续复制能力、激活侵袭和转移及诱导血管生成。在肿瘤中异常表达的 miRNA 被认为可通过作用于不同的靶基因影响一个或者几个上述的生物学过程。

1. 获得持续性生长信号和逃避生长抑制

细胞增殖是癌症最重要的标志，细胞增殖的异常是肿瘤发生的重要标志。实际上，细胞周期是由细胞内的程序和细胞外的信号分子共同控制，在促进和抑制细胞增殖之间达到平衡。细胞发生癌变时，细胞生长或分裂失控。近年的研究表明一些 miRNA 集成到多个关键细胞增殖途径通路，这些 miRNA 的失调导致癌细胞逃避生长抑制和（或）使癌细胞获得持续增殖信号。

一类转录因子 - E2F 家族是在细胞周期中调节细胞增殖的重要因素。一系列的研究表明，miRNA 参与 E2F 表达的调控。所述 E2F 家族中的分子 E2F1 在细胞周期 G_1 至 S 期转变的过程中诱导靶基因的转录，并且由于 E2F1 缺陷小鼠体内出现各种癌症所以其被定义为肿瘤抑制物。O'Donnell 等人发现 miR-17-92 簇被 c-Myc 激活后可抑制 E2F1 的翻译，考虑到 c-Myc 可直接调节 E2F1 的表达，miR-17-92 簇可以作为可能的正反馈环路制动措施，确保 E2F1 蛋白水平的急剧上升不会影响到 c-myc 的激活。miR-17-92 簇还被发现可以调节 E2F2 和 E2F3 的翻译，同时 E2F 的转录因子可以反过来促进 miR-17-92 簇的表达。miR-17-92 簇和 E2F 家族之间的调控环路可以使细胞周期保持稳定。在某些肿瘤中 miR-17-92 簇过表达时，这一环路失调促进细胞增殖。细胞周期可被不同的细胞周期蛋白、细胞周期蛋白激酶及他们的抑制剂调节，而这些周期蛋白可以被 miRNA 调控。其中 miR221/222 可以与 CDK 的抑制剂 p27Kip1 直接结合从而调控细胞周期。miR221/222 的异位表达可促进细胞增殖，从而抑制癌细胞在 G_1 细胞周期停滞。此外，

miR221/222 已被发现在多种人类肿瘤中上调，这表明 $p27^{Kip1}$ 是 miR221/222 调控是一个真正致癌途径。$p27^{Kip1}$，$P21^{CIP1}$ 和 $p16^{INK4a}$ 类似的也被 miRNA 如 miR – 663、miR – 302 家族和 miR – 24 调节。miR – 663 被发现在鼻咽癌中上调，并作为原癌基因，在体内外试验中通过直接靶向 $P21^{CIP1}$ 促进细胞 G_1/S 期之间的转化。

miRNA 不仅通过靶向细胞周期中的组分参与细胞增殖，而且可通过广泛调整多个信号通路从而调节细胞增殖。例如 miR – 486 在非小细胞肺癌显著下调，miR – 486 靶向（IGF1、IGF1R 和 $p85\alpha$.80）通过胰岛素生长受体（IGF）和 PI3K 信号传导途径的影响细胞增殖和迁移。

2. 抑制细胞死亡

凋亡逃逸是在肿瘤进展中被认为是由 miRNA 调节的另一显著标志。肿瘤细胞进化出多种策略来限制或规避凋亡。其中，p53 肿瘤抑制功能的丧失是最常见的一种方式。另一些逃避凋亡的方式包括抗凋亡因子的上调、促凋亡因子抑制和外源性配体诱导凋亡途径的抑制。参与抗凋亡的组件大多被 miRNA 抑制或激活。

已经鉴定出许多 p53 调节的 miRNA 参与调控 p53 基因的功能，在这些 miRNA 中有一些可以通过反馈调节方式调节 p53 的表达水平和活性。例如，Pichiorri 等人确定了在多发性骨髓瘤中，三个 miRNA（miR – 192、miR – 194 和 miR – 215）通过直接结合到 Mdm2 的 mRNA 3′非编码区使 Mdm2 的表达下降、使 p53 活化从而保护 p53，避免 p53 的降解。这些 miRNA 对 p53 基因有正性调节作用，而且它们的表达下调在多发性骨髓瘤发展中起到关键作用。还有另一种负反馈调节作用，miR – 122 通过直接靶向细胞周期蛋白 Gld2 和胞质聚腺苷酸化元件结合蛋白促进 p53 的活性，这为建立结合化疗和以 miRNA 为基础的肝细胞癌治疗方法提供了理论依据。

抗凋亡调节剂（Bcl - 2 和 Bcl - xL）和促凋亡因子（Bax、Bim 和 Puma）是一些 miRNA 的潜在目标，这些分子在细胞死亡中发挥重要作用。miR - 15a 和 miR - 16 - 1 在慢性淋巴细胞白血病中的表达显著下调且其表达与 Bcl - 2 的表达成反比。进一步的研究表明，这两个 miRNA 可抑制 Bcl - 2 的表达，诱导细胞凋亡。Denoyelle 等人发现在卵巢癌细胞中 miR - 491 - 5p 通过直接抑制 Bcl - xL 的表达并通过诱导 Bim 的积累诱导细胞凋亡。miRNA 也可通过调节参与外源性细胞凋亡途径中的分子，如 Fas 配体/ Fas 受体的表达从而抑制细胞死亡。miR - 21 在多种癌症中表达上调，miR - 21 可通过抑制 Apaf - 1 发挥作用，Apaf - 1 是外源性凋亡途径中一个关键引发剂，它是线粒体凋亡途径中的一个重要组成部分并可降低 Fas 的蛋白水平从而发挥抗凋亡功能。对 miR - 21 功能的进一步研究证实，miR - 21 的异位表达可保护由吉西他滨诱导的细胞凋亡。在 AML 中，Shaffiey 等人确定了 miR - 590 抑制 Fas 配体表达从而促进细胞存活。除了调节细胞凋亡配体的表达，miRNA 的失调也可通过调节死亡受体的表达抑制细胞死亡。例如，Razumilava 等人发现 miR - 25 在恶性胆管癌细胞中过表达，其能够通过靶向死亡受体 4（DR4）抑制肿瘤坏死因子相关凋亡通路中由配体介导的细胞凋亡。

3. 激活侵袭和转移

转移是一个复杂的、多步骤的、动态的生物学事件。上皮 - 间质转化（EMT）被认为在转移过程的早期和关键步骤中发挥重要的作用。上皮 - 间质转化主要特征是通过抑制 E - cadherin 从而使细胞黏附能力减弱或者激活促进细胞运动和侵袭相关的基因。EMT 被认为是由多种信号通路调节，如转化生长因子通路，这些关键转录因子包括 ZEB、SNAIL 以及 TWIST。

越来越多的证据表明，miRNA 在 EMT 和癌症转移中起重要作用。TGF－β 调控的 miRNA 被发现参与 TGF－β 信号通路以诱导 EMT 且在晚期恶性肿瘤中促进肿瘤细胞的转移。miR－155 是参与这一调节过程的 miRNA 之一。miR－155 在多种恶性肿瘤中过表达且在转录水平激活 TGF－β/SMAD4 信号。机制研究揭示了 miR－155 通过靶向的 RhoA GTP 酶促进 EMT。下调 miR－155 抑制 TGF－β 诱导的 EMT 和紧密连接的溶解，同时促进细胞迁移和侵袭。

　　TWIST 和 SNAIL 是另外两个关键转录因子，可通过调控某些 miRNA 的表达促进上皮细胞运动、侵袭和转移。例如，miR－10b 在转移性乳腺癌细胞中高表达，且正性调节细胞迁移和侵袭，miR－10b 可通过直接结合 TWIST 的 3′非编码区从而抑制其表达。此外，在非转移性 SUM149 和 SUM159 乳腺癌细胞系中 miR－10b 的异常表达可诱导恶性侵袭和微转移灶的形成。此外，miRNA 调控这些 EMT 因子的表达对于控制转移是至关重要的。例如，miR－203 在高转移性乳腺癌细胞中显著下调。miR－203 在乳腺癌细胞中通过抑制 SNAI2 抑制体内和体外肺转移和肿瘤细胞浸润，表明 SNAI2 和 miR－203 调节环路在 EMT 和肿瘤转移中具有重要作用。

　　其他参与调节转移过程的 miRNA 包括 miR－9 和 miR－212。miR－9 的表达依赖 c－Myc 和 n－Myc 的激活，这两者是通过直接与 miR－9－3 结合从而发挥作用的。miR－9 的表达水平与 MYCN 放大、肿瘤分级和转移状态密切相关。在患有转移性疾病的原发性乳腺肿瘤患者中，miR－9 的表达比无转移患者要高得多，这意味着的 miR－9 是转移过程中的潜在调节剂。Ma 等人确定了 miR－9 减少通过直接结合 E－钙黏蛋白的 3′非编码区从而抑制 E－钙黏蛋白的表达。miR－9 导致 E－钙黏蛋白下调的结果是 β－catenin 信号的激活从而触发下游致癌基因的表达，这导致肿瘤细胞运动性和侵袭性增加。进一步的实验证实在动物模型中，miR-9 的功能是通过 miRNA 的"海绵"功能发挥作用的，这意味着的 miR-9 的沉默可以作为乳腺癌预防转移一个新的治疗方法。

miR-210 是在缺氧过程中最重要的 miRNA。研究表明，在含氧量正常的人脐静脉内皮细胞中 miR-210 过表达可促进毛细管样结构的生成和 VEGF 依赖性细胞迁移的形成，相反，使用 miR-210 阻断剂可拮抗这些进程。最近的研究表明外泌体 miRNA 可以帮助调节肿瘤微环境。Umezu 等人发现 miR-135b 在耐低氧多发性骨髓瘤细胞的外泌体中过表达，在内皮细胞中抑制 factor-inhibiting HIF1 (FIH-1) 从而通过 HIF-FIH 信号通路促进内皮管道形成。由于启动子甲基化和杂合性缺失，在人类结直肠癌组织中 miR-212 显著下调。过表达的 miR-212 通过靶向 MnSOD 在体内抑制结直肠癌的迁移和侵袭并在体外抑制结直肠癌的肺转移。因此，miR-212 可以作为结直肠癌患者预后标志并且预测他们的生存时间，而且 miR-212 与 MnSOD 也可能是癌症治疗靶点。

4. 诱导血管生成

血管生成是从原有血管发展新生血管的高度协调过程，以满足肿瘤生长和转移所需的物质和氧气。与癌旁组织相比，肿瘤组织具有更低的氧浓度，缺氧对于癌细胞的发展和维持肿瘤微环境起到关键作用。缺氧诱导因子 (HIF) 是响应低氧的关键转录因子，HIF 可影响众多分子，其中就包括影响 miRNA 的表达。血管内皮生长因子 (VEGF) 是一个关键的血管生成因子，VEGF 通过直接结合上皮的受体使血管新生。因此，miRNA 靶向 HIF 或 VEGF 信号通路可能对血管生成产生显著影响。

在缺氧时，miR-210 是最稳定和显著诱导的 miRNA。两个独立的研究证明，在含氧量正常的人脐静脉内皮细胞中 miR-210 的过表达刺激毛细管样结构和 VEGF 依赖性的细胞迁移的形成。与此相反，miR-210 拮抗剂阻断这些进程。此外，miR-210 不仅通过靶向受体酪氨酸激酶的配体蛋白-A3，它是一种抗血管生成因子，也通过增强 VEGF 和 VEGF 受体-2（VEGFR2）的表达从而促进血管生成。

最近的研究表明，癌细胞外泌体中的 miRNA 可以帮助调节肿瘤微环境。Umezu 等人观察到耐低氧多发性骨髓瘤细胞的外泌体中 miR-135b 过表达，抑制内皮细胞因子 factor-inhibiting HIF1（FIH-1），从而通过 HIF-FIH 信号通路促进内皮管道形成。因此，外泌体重的 miR-135b 可以是用于控制多发性骨髓瘤的血管生成。

三、MicroRNA 与胃癌的侵袭和转移

MicroRNA 是由 22～24 个核苷酸组成的小的单链 RNA 分子，其作为癌基因或抑癌基因在肿瘤形成、浸润和转移过程中发挥重要作用。目前胃癌在所有恶性肿瘤中具有高发病率和死亡率的特点，并且缺乏早期特异性诊断标志物和有效的治疗手段。越来越多的研究表明 miRNA 能够调控参与胃癌发生、发展过程中的许多重要的肿瘤相关基因，从而调节胃癌的浸润和转移。

（一）miRNAs 抑制或者促进胃癌的转移

在胃癌组织中过表达 let-7f 可以直接结合肿瘤转移相关基因 MYH9 的 3′非编码区从而达到抑制肿瘤侵袭和转移的作用。对于肿瘤基因编码的胰岛素样生长因子 1 受体（IGF1R），miR-7通过直接结合 IGF1R 的 3′非编码区显著扭转上皮-间质转化进程并抑制胃癌体内、体外的侵袭和转移。癌基因

PDGFR 直接受 miR-34a 的调控，从而抑制胃癌细胞增殖、迁移和转移。miR-101 不仅能抑制增殖、侵袭和胃癌细胞的体外迁移，而且可以抑制胃癌体内的增殖能力。

在 80 个胃癌组织样品和 4 个胃癌细胞系中，miR-214 的表达水平比在正常组织和对照组细胞要低得多。miR-214 的表达水平与胃癌淋巴结转移和转移结节大小之间呈显著的负相关关系。在胃癌细胞系 SGC-7901 和 MKN-45 中，miR-214 异位表达可能降低的 miR-214 的肿瘤迁移和侵袭能力。下调 miR-214 可以在很大程度上刺激 MKN28、BGC-823 和 GES-1 细胞的增殖、迁移和侵袭。细胞集落刺激因子 1（CSF-1）是 miR-214 的靶基因中，而且低表达的 miR-214 可以促进胃癌细胞的增殖、迁移和侵袭，这些作用同 CSF-1 的表达呈负相关。

miR-9 的异常表达可促进胃癌细胞增殖、侵袭和转移。相比于正常组织，miR-9 往往在胃癌组织中有更低的表达水平。miR-10a 在胃癌细胞中的表达水平比正常胃黏膜高 10 倍。与早期胃癌患者相比，胃癌晚期患者出现淋巴结转移，表现出显著升高表达的 miR-10a。miR-20a 促进胃癌细胞的生长、迁移和侵袭。此外，它可以增强其对化疗药的抗性（顺铂和紫杉醇）。在胃肿瘤发生过程中，miR-20a 发挥作用主要通过调节 EGR2 信号传导途径实现的。miR-27 在调节胃癌转移中发挥重要的作且可能成为临床治疗的潜在靶点。高表达的 miR-27 促进 AGS 细胞的转移，机制主要是其通过激活 Wnt 通路促进 EMT 过程从而促进胃癌的转移。

（二）miRNA 与胃癌的淋巴结转移相关

淋巴结转移是恶性肿瘤的最常见转移途径，对患者的生存质量和预后产生严重影响。现已证实 miRNA 与恶性肿瘤的侵袭和转

移有密切关系。Wu 等人筛查胃癌组织和其邻近的正常组织发现
38 个 miRNA 分子的表达呈显著差异。进一步研究发现，5 个
miRNA分子与肿瘤淋巴转移相关，其中高表达的 miR – 195 水平与
低表达的 miR – 212 水平与淋巴转移密切相关。在胃癌中 miR –
650 与淋巴结转移及远处转移显著相关，miR – 650 的异位表达可
通过抑癌基因 ING4 调控促进胃肿瘤发生和胃癌细胞的增殖。

（三） miRNAs 与淋巴管生成

现在普遍认为淋巴管的形成是淋巴结转移的起始步骤，因
为它为肿瘤细胞提供了必要的转移途径。一项研究发现，在人
淋巴管内皮细胞中上调的 miR – 1236 的表达显著降低 VEGFR –
3 的表达而不是 VEGFR – 2 的表达，miR – 1236 的过表达可通过
影响淋巴管的新生从而削弱这些细胞的迁移和成管能力。在比
较参与淋巴管生成在正常淋巴管内皮细胞和那些来自 T – 241/
VEGF – C 的纤维肉瘤肿瘤转移模型中的淋巴管 miRNA 靶基因的
研究中。基因分型微阵列方法初步检测三个淋巴管生成相关的
基因，包括内皮细胞选择性黏附分子、TGF – β1/3 受体内皮糖
蛋白和血管生成相关受体，他们与淋巴管的生成密切相关。
miRNA 和淋巴管的关系正在成为肿瘤淋巴转移的研究热点。关
于 miRNA 及其靶基因的差异表达的进一步研究可能有助于找到
的癌症的新的诊断和治疗方法。

四、let – 7 家族与转移

MicroRNA let – 7 家族是较早发现的 microRNA 家族，目前已
发现的 let – 7 家族成员有 125 种，在人类中发现有 11 种 pre – let – 7

（hsa - let - 7a - 1，2，3、hsa - let - 7b、hsa - let - 7c、hsa - let -
7d、hsa - let - 7e、hsa - let - 7f - 1，2、hsa - let - 7g、hsa - let -
7i），共产生 8 种成熟的 let - 7。这些 let - 7 家族成员之间彼此基因
序列高度保守，功能相似。实验验证 let - 7 家族成员在不同肿瘤转
移中发挥不同的作用。

　　let - 7 家族在肺癌、卵巢癌、乳腺癌等多种肿瘤细胞中的表
达水平显著下调，而且其在肺癌和乳腺癌中的表达水平与患者
的生存时间呈正相关。let - 7 可通过与 RAS、HMGA2 和 c -
MYC 等多种基因靶向结合，负性调控其表达，从而调控肿瘤的
增殖、凋亡与分化，抑制肿瘤的发生与发展。

　　研究表明 let - 7 家族 miRNA 可通过多种靶分子和信号传导
通路抑制肿瘤转移。在人乳腺癌细胞中 let - 7 表达升高可减少
肝、肺转移瘤的发生率。随后的工作揭示了 let - 7 通过作用于
有利于转移的基因染色质重塑 HMGA2 蛋白和转录因子 BACH1
抑制细胞侵袭及其向骨转移。该 let - 7 调控网络通过抑制癌细
胞侵袭的细胞内在表型抑制转移。let - 7 直接靶向 HMGA2 和
BACH1 导致一系列促进侵袭基因的转录抑制。let - 7 可被 LIN -
28 调控，这影响了 let - 7 的 miRNA 前体从而最终促进转移。
RKIP，一个 LIN - 28 间接作用靶点，通过 let - 7 上调抑制肿瘤
的转移。

　　let - 7 可以靶向 Rsf - 1 的上游激动剂 RAS，从而出现正反
馈回路调控肿瘤的侵袭和转移。引人注意的是，Yu 等人发现在
乳腺癌干细胞中 let - 7 上调，let - 7 通过靶向 H - RAS 和
HMGA2，H - RAS 和 HMGA2 随着 let - 7 过表达而下调。然而，
H - RAS 和 HMGA2 之间的生物学功能差异显著：在肿瘤干细胞
中沉默 H - RAS 导致乳腺癌细胞自我更新能力增强，但其对分
化没有影响。相比之下，沉默 HMGA2 可增强细胞分化，但不影
响自我更新。癌症干细胞具有无限自我更新的能力，并且可以

分化成多种细胞类型，使肿瘤细胞能够在治疗后重新增殖而且具有远处转移的能力。有趣的是，MYC 可在转录后水平被 let-7 调节，但它也可以通过抑制 RNA polymerase-Ⅱ阻止 let-7 前体的转录从而控制 let-7（或其他 microRNA）的表达。

Han 等发现在胃癌中 let-7b 可作为肿瘤抑制因素阻止胃癌细胞的侵袭和转移，let-7b 可以直接结合 ING1 的 3′非编码区从而发挥其抑制胃癌侵袭和转移的作用，而且比较胃癌组织和与其对应的癌旁组织发现胃癌组织中 let-7b 的表达低于癌旁组织。Subramanian 等人发现肿瘤抑制 microRNA let-7i 通过内源性表达 p53 基因的突变在多种细胞系表达下调。在乳腺癌患者中，显著下降的 let-7i 水平与 p53 基因的错义突变相关。染色质免疫沉淀和启动子荧光素酶检测发现 let-7i 通过 P63 从而作用于突变的 p53 从而介导转录。在 p53 突变的细胞中，let-7i 可通过抑制多种癌基因，包括 E2F5、LIN28B、MYC 和 NRAS 网络显著促进迁移、侵袭和转移。

Ghanbari R. 等人对 8 例 CRC 患者和四个健康受试者的血浆和粪便样品进行 miRNA 表达谱芯片分析。与健康受试者相比，在患者血浆和粪便样品中有七个低表达 microRNA。然后，我们通过对更大的一组 51 例患者血浆和 26 例健康受试者血浆和粪便样本进行定量逆转录聚合酶链反应分析。通过微阵列分析发现 let-7a-5p 和 let-7f-5p 的表达在 CRC 患者的粪便和血浆样品中显著降低。在 CRC 患者血浆和粪便样品中低表达的 let-7a-5p 和 let-7f-5p 可作为早期检测结直肠癌潜在的非侵入性分子标志物。

五、FNDC3B 介导 microRNA let - 7f - 5p 抑制胃癌转移的研究

近年来，很多测序结果显示 microRNA 在胃癌及其癌旁组织中的表达存在差异。这些研究为 miRNAs 在胃癌形成过程中发挥重要作用提供了有力依据。通过文献回顾发现，Ueda 等利用 miRNA 微阵列分析了两个独立胃癌患者组共 353 份胃癌组织样本，根据 Lauren 分型和胃癌浸润深度、转移和分期，通过多变量回归分析，以确定 miRNA 在胃癌不同阶段的表达模式。研究发现，let - 7f 在胃癌转移组织中的表达水平下降，且与胃癌的浸润深度、淋巴结转移和临床分期呈负相关。为了研究 microRNA let - 7f - 5p 的功能，我们选用一对由本实验室筛选并验证的胃癌高低转移细胞系 MKN28M 和 MKN28NM，在这对高低转移细胞系中通过实时荧光定量 PCR 实验检测 let - 7f - 5p 的表达情况，进一步通过 transwell 实验验证 let - 7f - 5p 可抑制胃癌的迁移和侵袭。随后我们通过结合四个生物学预测软件（Targetscan、CLIP - Seq、miRanda 及 miRDB）来预测 let - 7f - 5p 的靶基因，在这些靶基因中我们认为 FNDC3B 十分有可能是 let - 7f - 5p 的靶基因，通过双荧光素报告基因实验我们证实 FNDC3B 为 let - 7f - 5p 的靶基因。

FNDC3B 属于 FN3 家族，FNDC3B 为 Fibronectin type Ⅲ domain containing，即纤连蛋白Ⅲ型结构域，包括 157 个分子，其中有我们熟悉的在 IGF1R、ROBO1 等。本实验室的前期研究发现 miR - 7 可通过抑制 IGF1R 从而抑制胃癌的转移，miR - 218 可通过 Robo1 - slit 通路抑制胃癌的转移。在 FN3 家族中，FNDC

有九个分子，即 FNDC1、FNDC2、FNDC3A、FNDC3B、FNDC4、FNDC5、FNDC7、FNDC8 和 FNDC9，其中 FNDC3 有两个亚型，即 FNDC3A 和 FNDC3B，由于这两个分子的相关研究较少，目前认为它们在生理过程中发挥的作用是：FNDC3A 在精子形成过程中介导精子细胞与支持细胞粘连，FNDC3B 可能对脂肪形成有正性调节作用。在癌症的发生、发展中，FNDC3B 主要是通过被 miR - 143 调控而发挥作用的，在肝癌细胞中 FNDC3B 通过 NF - κB - miR - 143 - FNDC3B 轴来调节肝癌的转移；在前列腺癌细胞中也可通过 miR - 143 - FNDC3B 轴来调节前列腺癌的转移。但是在胃癌中 FNDC3B 所发挥的作用还有待进一步研究。

（刘　刚）

参考文献

[1] Chen W, Zheng R, Baade PD, et al. Cancer statistics in China, 2015. CA Cancer J Clin, 2016, 66：115 - 132.

[2] Thrumurthy SG, Chaudry MA, Hochhauser D, et al. The diagnosis and management of gastric cancer. BMJ, 2013, 347：f6367.

[3] Sun Y, Ma L. The emerging molecular machinery and therapeutic targets of metastasis. Trends Pharmacol Sci, 2015, 36：349 - 359.

[4] Nguyen DX, Joan M. Genetic determinants of cancer metastasis. Nat Rev Genet, 2007, 8：341 - 352.

[5] Raza U, Zhang JD, Sahin Ö. MicroRNAs：master regulators of drug resistance, stemness, and metastasis. J Mol Med, 2014, 92：321 - 336.

[6] Ling H, Fabbri M, Calin GA. MicroRNAs and other non - coding RNAs as targets for anticancer drug development. Nat Rev Drug Discov, 2013, 12：847 - 865.

[7] Lin Z, Jia H, Nuo Y, et al. microRNAs exhibit high frequency genomic alterations in human cancer. Proc Natl Acad Sci USA, 2006, 103：9136 - 9141.

[8]　Zhao X, He L, Li T, et al. SRF expedites metastasis and modulates the epithelial to mesenchymal transition by regulating miR – 199a – 5p expression in human gastric cancer. Cell Death Differ, 2014, 21; 1900 – 1913.

[9]　Raver – Shapira N, Marciano E, Meiri E, et al. Transcriptional activation of miR – 34a contributes to p53 – mediated apoptosis. Mol Cell, 2007, 26; 731 – 743.

[10]　Merritt WM, Lin YG, Han LY, et al. Dicer,Drosha, and outcomes in patients with ovarian cancer. N Engl J Med, 2008, 359; 2641 – 2650.

[11]　Francesco F, Serena R, Giuseppe Z, et al. Epigenetic silencing of themyelopoiesis regulator microRNA – 223 by the AML1/ETO oncoprotein. Cancer Cell, 2007, 12; 457 – 466.

[12]　Yoshimasa S, Gangning L, Gerda E, et al. Specific activation of microRNA – 127 with downregulation of the proto – oncogene BCL6 by chromatin – modifying drugs in human cancer cells. Cancer Cell, 2006, 9;435 – 443.

[13]　Amaia L, Calin GA, Alberto V, et al. A microRNA DNA methylation signature for human cancer metastasis. Proc Natl Acad Sci, 2008, 105; 13556 – 13561.

[14]　Lehmann U,Hasemeier B, Christgen M, et al. Epigenetic inactivation of microRNA gene hsa – mir – 9 – 1 in human breast cancer. J Pathol, 2008, 214; 17 – 24.

[15]　Douglas H, Weinberg RA. Hallmarks of cancer; the next generation. Cell, 2011, 144; 646 – 674.

[16]　Woods K, Thomson JM, Hammond SM. Direct regulation of an oncogenic micro – RNA cluster by E2F transcription factors. J Biol Chem, 2007, 282;2130 – 2134.

[17]　Lorimer IAJ. Regulation of p27Kip1 bymiRNA 221/222 in glioblastoma. Cell Cycle, 2009, 8; 2005 – 2009.

[18]　Dasa D, Marek M, Tomas B, et al. MicroRNAs regulate p21 (Waf1/Cip1) protein expression and the DNA damage response in human embryonic stem cells. Stem Cells, 2012, 30; 1362 – 1372.

[19]　Yi C, Wang Q, Wang L, et al. MiR – 663, amicroRNA targeting p21

(WAF1/CIP1), promotes the proliferation and tumorigenesis of nasopharyngeal carcinoma. Oncogene, 2012, 31: 4421 - 4433.

[20] Yong P, Yuntao D, Charles H, et al. Insulin growth factor signaling is regulated bymicroRNA - 486, an underexpressed microRNA in lung cancer. Proce Natl Acad Sci USA, 2013, 110: 15043 - 15048.

[21] Li C, Hashimi SM, Good DA, et al. Apoptosis and microRNA aberrations in cancer. Clin Exp Pharmacol Physiol, 2012, 39: 739 - 746.

[22] Flavia P, Sung - Suk S, Alberto R, et al. Downregulation of p53 - inducible microRNAs 192, 194, and 215 impairs the p53/MDM2 autoregulatory loop in multiple myeloma development. Cancer Cell, 2010, 18: 367 - 381.

[23] Burns DM, Andrea DA, Stephanie N, et al. CPEB and two poly(A) polymerases control miR - 122 stability and p53 mRNA translation. Nature, 2011, 473: 105 - 108.

[24] Denoyelle C, Lambert B, Meryet - Figuière M, et al. miR - 491 - 5p - induced apoptosis in ovarian carcinoma depends on the direct inhibition of both BCL - XL and EGFR leading to BIM activation. Cell Death Dis, 2014, 5: e1445.

[25] Peng W, Liping Z, Juan Z, et al. The serum miR - 21 level serves as a predictor for thechemosensitivity of advanced pancreatic cancer, and miR - 21 expression confers chemoresistance by targeting FasL. Mol Oncol, 2013, 7:334 - 345.

[26] Nataliya R, Bronk SF, Smoot RL, et al. miR - 25 targets TNF - related apoptosis inducing ligand (TRAIL) death receptor - 4 and promotes apoptosis resistance in cholangiocarcinoma. Hepatology, 2012, 55:465 - 475.

[27] Kalluri R, Weinberg RA. Kalluri R, et al. The basics of epithelial - mesenchymal transition. J Clin Invest, 2009, 119: 1420 - 1428.

[28] William K, Hua Y, Lili H, et al. MicroRNA - 155 is regulated by the transforming growth factor beta/Smad pathway and contributes to epithelial cell plasticity by targeting RhoA. Mol Cell Biol, 2008, 28: 6773 - 6784.

[29] Li M, Julie TF, Weinberg RA. Tumour invasion and metastasis initiated bymicroRNA - 10b in breast cancer. Nature, 2007, 449: 682 - 688.

[30] Ding X, Park SI, McCauley LK, et al. Signaling between transforming growth factor β (TGF - β) and transcription factor SNAI2 represses expre ssion ofmicroRNA miR - 203 to promote epithelial - mesenchymal transition and tumor metastasis. J Biol Chem, 2013, 288:10241 - 10253.

[31] Ma L, Young JH, Pan E, et al. miR - 9, a MYC/MYCN - activatedmicroRNA, regulates E - cadherin and cancer metastasis. Nat Cell Biol, 2010, 12: 247 - 256.

[32] Almeida MI, Reis RM, Calin GA. MYC - microRNA - 9 - metastasis connection in breast cancer. Cell Res, 2010, 20: 603 - 604.

[33] Lou YL, Guo F, Liu F, et al. miR - 210 activates notch signaling pathway in angiogenesis induced by cerebral ischemia. Mol Cell Biochem, 2012, 370:45 - 51.

[34] Tomohiro U, Hiroko T, Kenko A, et al. Exosomal miR - 135b shed from hypoxic multiple myeloma cells enhances angiogenesis by targeting factor - inhibiting HIF - 1. Blood, 2014, 124: 3748 - 3757.

[35] Meng X, Wu J, Pan C, et al. Genetic and epigenetic down - regulation ofmicroRNA - 212 promotes colorectal tumor metastasis via dysregulation of MnSOD. Gastroenterology, 2013, 145: 426 - 436. e1 - 6.

[36] Liu F, Lou YL, Wu J, et al. Upregulation of microRNA - 210 regulates renal angiogenesis mediated by activation of VEGF signaling pathway under ischemia/perfusion injury in vivo and in vitro. Kidney Blood Press Res, 2012, 35: 182 - 191.

[37] Lin S, Gregory RI. MicroRNA biogenesis pathways in cancer. Nat Rev Cancer, 2015, 15: 321 - 333.

[38] Liang S, He L, Zhao X, et al. MicroRNA let - 7f inhibits tumor invasion and metastasis by targeting MYH9 in human gastric cancer. PLoS One, 2011, 6: e18409.

[39] Zhao X, Dou W, He L, et al. MicroRNA - 7 functions as an anti - metastatic microRNA in gastric cancer by targeting insulin - like growth factor - 1 receptor. Oncogene, 2013, 32: 1363 - 1372.

[40] Wang HJ, Ruan HJ, He XJ, et al. MicroRNA - 101 is down - regulated

in gastric cancer and involved in cell migration and invasion. Eur J Cancer, 2010, 46: 2295 – 2303.

[41] Tsai KW, Liao YL, Wu CW, et al. Aberranthypermethylation of miR – 9 genes in gastric cancer. Epigenetics, 2011, 6: 1189 – 1197.

[42] Chen W, Tang Z, Sun Y, et al. miRNA expression profile in primary gastric cancers and paired lymph node metastases indicates that miR – 10a plays a role in metastasis from primary gastric cancer to lymph nodes. Exp Ther Med, 2012, 3: 351 – 356.

[43] Li X, Zhang Z, Yu M, et al. Involvement of miR – 20a in promoting gastric cancer progression by targeting early growth response 2 (EGR2). Int J Mol Sci, 2013, 14: 16226 – 16239.

[44] Zhang Z, Liu S, Shi R, et al. miR – 27 promotes human gastric cancer cell metastasis by inducing epithelial – to – mesenchymal transition. Cancer Genet, 2011, 204: 486 – 491.

[45] Zhang X, Zhu W, Zhang J, et al. MicroRNA – 650 targets ING4 to promote gastric cancer tumorigenicity. Biochem Biophys Res Commun, 2010, 395: 275 – 280.

[46] Jones D, Li Y, He Y, et al. Mirtron microRNA – 1236 inhibits VEGFR – 3 signaling during inflammatory lymphangiogenesis. Arterioscler Thromb Vasc Biol, 2012, 32: 633 – 642.

[47] Steven C, Daniel R, Dilair B, et al. A novel gene expression profile in lymphatics associated with tumor growth and nodal metastasis. Cancer Res, 2008, 68: 7293 – 7303.

[48] Yang J, Zhou F, Xu T, et al. Analysis of sequence variations in 59 microRNAs in hepatocellular carcinomas. Mutat Res, 2008, 638: 205 – 209.

[49] Dangi – Garimella S, Yun J, Eves E, et al. Raf kinase inhibitory protein suppresses a metastasis signalling cascade involving LIN28 and let – 7. EMBO J, 2009, 28: 347 – 358.

[50] Yun J, Frankenberger CA, Kuo WL, et al. Signalling pathway for RKIP and let – 7 regulates and predicts metastatic breast cancer. EMBO J, 2011, 30: 4500 – 4514.

[51] Yu F, Yao H, Zhu P, et al. Let - 7 regulates self renewal andtumorigenicity of breast cancer cells. Cell, 2007, 131: 1109 - 1123.

[52] Agnieszka R, Heiko F, Lena S, et al. A feedback loop comprising lin - 28 and let - 7 controls pre - let - 7 maturation during neural stem - cell commitment. Nat Cell Biol, 2008, 10: 987 - 993.

[53] Han X, Chen Y, Yao N, et al. MicroRNA let - 7b suppresses human gastric cancer malignancy by targeting ING1. Cancer Gene Ther,2015,22:122 - 129.

[54] Subramanian M, Francis P, Bilke S, et al. A mutant p53/let - 7i - axis - regulated gene network drives cell migration, invasion and metastasis. Oncogene, 2015,34:1094 - 1104.

[55] Ghanbari R,Mosakhani N, Sarhadi VK,et al. Simultaneous underexpression of let - 7a - 5p and let - 7f - 5p microRNAs in plasma and stool samples from early stage colorectal carcinoma. Biomark Cancer, 2015, 7:39 - 48.

[56] Tetsuya U, Stefano V, Hiroshi O, et al. Relation between microRNA expression and progression and prognosis of gastric cancer: a microRNA expression analysis. Lancet Oncol, 2010, 11: 136 - 146.

[57] Tie J, Pan Y, Zhao L,et al. MiR - 218 inhibits invasion and metastasis of gastric cancer by targeting theRobo1 receptor. PLoS Genet,2010,6:108 - 117.

[58] Zhang X, Liu S, Hu T, et al. Up - regulatedmicroRNA - 143 transcribed by nuclear factor kappa B enhances hepatocarcinoma metastasis by repressing fibronectin expression. Hepatology, 2009, 50: 490 - 499.

[59] Fan X, Xu C, Deng W, et al. Up - regulatedmicroRNA - 143 in cancer stem cells differentiation promotes prostate cancer cells metastasis by modulating FNDC3B expression. BMC Cancer, 2013, 13: 1 - 11.

第五章
上皮间充质转化与胃癌转移

一、肿瘤转移的研究现状

恶性肿瘤是一类严重危害人类健康的疾病，2012年全球新发肿瘤病例约14 100 000例，死亡病例数约8 200 000例，其中超过30%的病例发生在中国。未发生转移的肿瘤经手术和放射线治疗往往能得到较好的控制，然而大多数肿瘤起病隐匿，通常发现时已处于进展期并伴有淋巴结或远处转移。而对于转移肿瘤通常采用化学、激素和放射线等姑息疗法，有些研究表明尽管具有统计学上的差异，这对生存预后仅起到微小的作用——实体肿瘤中大约90%的死亡仍然来自转移。

肿瘤转移是指肿瘤细胞从原发部位，经淋巴、血液循环系统或体腔等途径，到达其他部位继续生长。这一生物学级联事件可大致分为以下几个步骤：局部浸润，进入淋巴管或血液循环系统，抵御免疫系统攻击并存活下来，在远端组织定植并形成继发肿瘤灶。每个步骤都是多因素调控，多分子参与的复杂过程。

（一）局部浸润

首先，由于DNA突变，染色质重排以及表观遗传学改变，肿瘤细胞获得异质性，为筛选出有利于其生存的特性提供了先决条件。随后在肿瘤微环境的作用压力下筛选出具有运动侵袭、抗凋亡、分解基底膜及细胞外基质能力的肿瘤细胞。参与其中的微环境因素包括细胞外基质、基底膜、活性氧、有限的营养物质和氧气以及免疫系统的攻击。肿瘤组织缺氧是一种强有力的筛选压力，可以促进肿瘤细胞的浸润生长和抗凋亡能力。低氧环境可增强缺氧诱导因子 1（HIF - 1）转录复合体的稳定性，从而致使促血管生成、细胞存活和侵袭相关分子的表达增加、转移复发以及生存时间的降低。

另外，微环境中的巨噬细胞分为 M1 型和 M2 型。M1 型巨噬细胞参与促炎反应，在免疫系统防卫中发挥关键效应；而肿瘤的低氧环境可募集巨噬细胞并诱导分化为具有肿瘤促进功能的 M2 型。目前许多研究已证明肿瘤相关巨噬细胞（TAM）通常属于 M2 型，可增强肿瘤细胞的侵袭转移能力。在乳腺癌，TAM 细胞分泌的 EGF 可提高肿瘤细胞集落刺激因子 CSF - 1 的表达水平，同时肿瘤细胞分泌的 CSF - 1 可促进 TAM 表达 EGF，以此形成的正反馈环路可明显增强肿瘤细胞的侵袭转移能力。在肿瘤转移前沿，TAM 是蛋白水解酶的主要来源，如半胱氨酸组织蛋白酶能降解 I 型胶原并活化间质胶原酶原，参与到肿瘤的浸润转移。

（二）脉管运输

然后，肿瘤细胞需要突破相关的脉管系统以运输至远处器官，这个过程需要建立新生血管并且介导恶性肿瘤逃脱或抑制宿主免疫系统。上述的 TAM 不仅可以促进肿瘤细胞的侵袭转移能力，亦对肿瘤转移进行着多方面的支持——促进血管生成、抑制抗肿瘤免疫反应，以及促进肿瘤细胞穿出血管然后定植。近期，多光子活体成像技术应用于观察肿瘤细胞播散时 TAM 和肿瘤的相互作用，结果显示 TAM 主要定位于肿瘤外围基质，而肿瘤深部的 TAM 数目较少，通常分布在血管周围协助肿瘤细胞进入血液循环。

此外，骨髓来源的抑制性细胞（MDSC）在肿瘤生成和浸润过程中被动员，打破由树突状细胞、活化 T 细胞、M1 型巨噬细胞和 NK 细胞组成的免疫监视系统，并发挥促血管生成作用。MDSC 可促进肿瘤进展这一观点得到了临床数据的支持，研究显示外周血中 MDSC 的含量与患者肿瘤分期和转移瘤负荷呈正相关。因为 MDSC 是分化异常导致的一类不成熟骨髓细胞，它们包含了不同成熟度和可塑性的细胞亚群。有研究将单核细胞来源的 MDSC 重编程可使其丧失 T 细胞抑制能力，产生 Th1 细胞因子，并分化成巨噬细胞，发挥肿瘤抑制作用，具有良好的治疗潜力。

（三）远处定植

不同类型的肿瘤通常只会扩散到特异的器官，早在 1889 年，Stephen Paget 便据此提出经典的"种子和土壤"学说。为解释 Paget 学说，有研究表明，在转移播散之前，肿瘤会分泌可促进预转移微环境形成的因子，预转移微环境具有大量骨髓源性细胞，成纤维细胞和促肿瘤的分泌蛋白及细胞因子，为肿瘤转移提供适宜的环境。Erler 等通过一项关于乳腺癌的研究发现，低氧诱导因子（HIF）信号通路的主要靶点赖氨酰氧化酶（LOX）的表达可促进肺部骨髓细胞的募集以及随后的肿瘤细胞定植，然而抑制肿瘤细胞 LOX 的表达，可阻止预转移微环境以及乳腺癌肺转移灶的形成。此外，有研究希望检测肿瘤缺氧会对预转移微环境产生怎样的影响。Sceneay 将低氧条件下培养乳腺癌细胞收集的培养基注射到小鼠体内，尽管没有注射任何肿瘤细胞，仍然可以观察到骨髓源性细胞和细胞毒性减弱的 NK 细胞浸润到肺部组织。这些研究均论证了骨髓源性细胞在预转移位点的预测和导向起到关键作用，并阐明了原发部位和转移器官之间交流的重要性。

我们已经知道，旁分泌的细胞因子和它们的受体在肿瘤微环境细胞间的信号传递中起到十分关键的作用。近期，作为细胞间信号传递的另一种模式，外泌体受到广泛研究。近期，Peinado 等研究人员探索了黑色素瘤来源的外泌体在原位肿瘤形成和转移中的作用。他们把高侵袭性黑色素瘤细胞系 B16 - F10 来源的外泌体注射入老鼠体内发现，这些外泌体选择性地分布在 B16 - F10 转移亲和器官肺、骨髓、肝、脾的组织间隙中，同时增加了该处的血管通透性，提示我们外泌体可以决定转移器官取向。而且将 B16 - F10 接种于小鼠皮下后，分别注射 B16 - F10 或低侵袭性 B16 - F1 细胞系来源的外泌体，观察到肺部转移瘤负荷前者是后者的 240 倍，说明外泌体可以决定转移潜能。其机制是通过 B16 - F10 来源的含有受体酪氨酸激酶 MET 的外泌体将MET 转移至骨髓祖细胞，对骨髓祖细胞实行重编程，使其向促血管生成表型转化，从而提高原发部位肿瘤的转移能力。

二、上皮间充质转化是肿瘤转移的重要机制

EMT 是指上皮细胞通过特定程序转化为具有间充质表型细胞的生物学过程。Elizabeth Hay 最早在 20 世纪 80 年代早期观察到鸡胚原条中的上皮 - 间充质形态学变化这一现象。近年来，人们发现除胚胎发育外，EMT 还参与到创口修复、组织纤维化和肿瘤进展等多种病理生理过程。上皮细胞通过紧密连接、黏着连接和桥粒建立规则紧密排列和顶 - 低端极性，并由基底膜将之与周围组织隔开；相反，间充质细胞在细胞外基质和结缔

组织中松散分布。在转移早期，上皮细胞通过 EMT 过程，丧失细胞黏附和细胞极性并获得运动和侵袭能力，使肿瘤细胞得以向周围浸润和播散，当肿瘤细胞随循环系统到达转移组织，再经间充质上皮转化（MET）恢复上皮细胞特性，以利于肿瘤细胞在转移组织处的黏附定植。

（一）上皮细胞连接和细胞极性丧失

细胞表面蛋白复合体形成的细胞间连接对于维持上皮完整性起到必要的保障作用。细胞间连接包括近顶端的紧密连接，侧面的黏着连接、桥粒及散在的缝隙链接。EMT 发生之时，细胞间连接发生解体，伴随有连接蛋白的转位或者降解。其中紧密连接是由跨膜蛋白 claudin 和 occludin，及膜外周蛋白 ZO 构成；黏着连接指 E－钙黏素通过连环蛋白（catenin）与肌动蛋白相连；桥粒指跨膜蛋白 E－钙黏素通过附着蛋白与中间纤维相连接。Ohtani 等通过免疫组化检测了紧密连接蛋白 claudin－4、occludin 和 ZO－1 在正常胃黏膜组织和胃癌组织中的表达，occludin 和 ZO－1 在未分化胃癌中表达显著降低，claudin－4 在未分化、发生淋巴结和腹膜转移的胃癌中呈低表达，提示 claudin－4 对胃癌侵袭转移潜能的降低发挥重要作用。E－钙黏素在胞膜处发生断裂后降解，因此与 E－钙黏素相互连接的 β－catenin 则处于游离状态，接着被分解或入核发挥转录作用。类似的是，随着 E－钙黏素表达水平的降低，p120－catenin 亦在细胞核内积聚参与基因转录。

E－钙黏素表达下调造成的黏着连接解体是 EMT 发生的一个标志性事件。Snail 蛋白、碱性螺旋环螺旋（bHLH）转录因子和 Zeb 蛋白是最常见的 E－钙黏蛋白转录抑制因子，这些转录因子在转录水平和转录后水平均可被调节，进一步影响 E－钙黏蛋白及 EMT。据此，形成了以 E - 钙黏蛋白及其转录因子为中心的巨大的 EMT 调控网络。TGF - β 通过 SMAD3 依赖的信号通路一方面可直接诱导 Snail1 的表达，另外又可促进转录因子 MRTF 的表达对 Snail2（Slug）起到间接增强的作用。在细胞培养中，表皮生长因子（EGF）不仅诱导 E - 钙黏蛋白的内吞作用，同时促进 Snail1 和 Twist 的表达转录抑制 E - 钙黏蛋白，进一步促进肿瘤细胞的迁移。此外，Notch 通路在 EMT 过程中亦扮演者重要的角色，在肺腺癌细胞中 Notch1 的抑制可部分逆转 EMT 从而降低细胞的侵袭转移能力。

上皮细胞连接蛋白编码基因的表达抑制通常伴随促进间充质黏着蛋白编码基因的激活。而下调的 E - 钙黏素被上调的 N - 钙黏素所平衡，导致"钙黏素转换"，通过这种转换，发生 EMT 的细胞失去与上皮细胞的联系，而通过 N - 钙黏素间相互作用获得与间充质细胞的亲和性，但是 N - 钙黏素间相互作用较上皮细胞间的黏着连接力量减弱，可促进细胞的迁移与侵袭。N - 钙黏素可通过 α - catenin 和 β - catenin 与细胞骨架相连，他还和 p120 - catenin、受体酪氨酸激酶（RTK）如血小板源生长因子（PDGF）及成纤维细胞生长因子受体（FGFR）相互作用并发挥调节功能。此外 EMT 亦可激活神经细胞黏着分子（NCAM），其通过与 N - 钙黏素相互作用来调节 RTK 的活性。

此外，通过与基底膜的连接以及极性复合体的参与，上皮细胞表现出顶 - 底极性。PAR（由 PAR6、PAR3 和 aPKC 蛋白组成）和 Crumbs（由 CRB、PALS1 和 PATJ 蛋白组成）复合体负责上皮细胞顶端区域的形成，Scribble（由 SCRIB、DLG 和 LGL 蛋白组成）复合体负责基底部区域的形成。上述极性相关复合体与细胞连接相关复合体存在紧密联系，因此 E - 钙黏素的表达缺失可阻止 SCRIB 与侧面胞膜相互作用，并且有研究发现 EMT 的发生可以使极性复合体相关蛋白，如 CRB3 和 LGL2 表达降低，均可导致细胞极性的降低。

（二） 细胞外基质重塑

细胞外基质的重塑和细胞与基质间的相互作用的改变是 EMT 发生、发展的必要条件。整合素的主要生物学功能表现为介导细胞与细胞外基质的黏附以及信号转导。在 EMT 过程中，其通常出现异常高表达，或新型整合素的合成。这些异常表达的整合素经内外信号转导，一方面影响肿瘤细胞与细胞外基质的黏附，使得细胞具有更强的侵袭性；另一方面通过与其配体结合，向细胞内传递信号介导 FAK/STAT、FAK/Ras/MAPK、FAK/PI3K 等多条通路的信号转导，从而影响转移在内的多种恶性表型。EMT 过程中，整合素 β_4 的编码基因发生表观遗传学沉默，从而导致介导上皮细胞与基底膜连接的整合素 $\alpha_6\beta_4$ 表达下调；整合素 $\alpha_5\beta_1$ 的表达升高可增强细胞与纤连蛋白间的黏着，从而促进细胞迁移。在 AGS 胃癌细胞中，使用整合素 $\alpha v\beta_3$ 的中和性抗体，可以阻断 NF - κB 的激活及下游 COX - 2 的基因表达，进而降低细胞的侵袭性。Takatsuki 等研究人员首先将 NUGC - 4 胃癌细胞细胞系用整合素 α_2 或 α_3 亚基的抗体进行孵育，然后接种到 BALB/c nu/nu 小鼠腹腔内，结果显示抗 α_3 整合素抗体处理组、α_2 整合素抗体处理组与对照组产生的腹膜结节数依次减少，并且在 β_1 亚基阳性、α_2 和 α_3 亚基阴性的白血病细胞中导入整合素 α_2 和 α_3 的 cDNA，发现转染整合素 α_3 的细胞与单层腹膜间皮细胞的附着较转染整合素 α_2 和阴性对照的细胞更加牢固，说明整合素 $\alpha_3\beta_1$ 在介导胃癌细胞与腹膜最初的附着及腹膜转移的形成中扮演关键的角色。此外临床标本中检测整合素 β_3 的表达与胃癌组织的血管密度、浸润程度和淋巴结转移密切相关。目前整合素的拮抗剂 cilengitide 已进入多种肿瘤的临床试验中，加上整合素参与到胃癌转移级联事件的多个阶段，因此 cilengitide 亦有望运用于胃癌临床试验。

其次，细胞外基质的降解主要由基质金属蛋白酶（MMP）所介导。在正常组织中，MMP 的功能通过转录或转录后机制得以很好的控制，然而，肿瘤细胞演变出多种途径打破这一控制来增强 MMP 的功能。MMP 共分为 23 种，其中他们共享的结构是前导肽、催化区和血色素结合蛋白样的羧端结构域。MMP 最初产生时由于前导肽的半胱氨酸残基和催化结构域的锌离子相结合，导致其处于无活性状态。因此目前有关 MMP 的研究主要集中在 MMP 的表达和活性调控。例如在非小细胞肺癌中，MMP9 的表达可通过 NF－κB 通路的激活被增强；在口腔恶性肿瘤中，促癌的 miR－196 通过 NME4－JNK 抑制 TIMP1。TIMP1 是一种能特异性抑制 MMP 活性的低分子量蛋白质，最终激活 MMP1 和 MMP9 促进肿瘤的侵袭。除此之外，MMP 可靶向作用于一些跨膜蛋白，导致例如 E－钙黏素胞外区域的释放，和随之发生的黏着连接的缺失。

（三）细胞骨架重排

经历 EMT 的细胞会发生细胞骨架重排，使细胞得以延伸和定向移动，主要通过肌动蛋白富集的膜突起来实现，包括板状伪足及其末端刺突样的丝状伪足。这个过程中主要由小 G 蛋白 RHO 调节肌动蛋白动力学并控制肌动蛋白重排。RHO 具有 GTP（鸟苷三磷酸）酶活性，与 GTP 结合时为活化形式，而当 GTP 水解为 GDP 时则回复到非活化状态。细胞中存在着一些调控小 G 蛋白活性的调节因子，如鸟苷酸交换因子（guanine nucleotide exchange factor，GEF）可增强小 G 蛋白的活性，GTP 酶活化蛋白（GTPase activating protein，GAP）可降低小 G 蛋白活性。

RHO 家族由 Rho、Rac 和 Cdc42 三类分子构成。其中活化的 Rac 和 Cdc42 可诱导丝状伪足和板状伪足的形成，促进细胞向前延伸，而 Rho 往往被认为起到诱导细胞运动尾部收缩的作用，三者相互协调，共同促进细胞的运动。

（四） EMT 作为肿瘤转移机制存在的问题

尽管 EMT 在肿瘤转移中的作用已经得到广泛研究，越来越多的证据表明 EMT 作用参与了肿瘤转移，而且已经有研究以此为靶点进行新药的开发。但这一理论始终存在争议，主要是因为该理论还没有真正从人体肿瘤转移标本中获得支持，以及无法通过在体实验对短暂性和可逆性 EMT 过程造成的表型进行观察。近日，Gao 等研究人员在自发性乳腺癌肺转移的小鼠模型中，利用间充质细胞特异的 Cre 介导的荧光标记开关建立了一个 EMT 跟踪系统。他们发现，在上皮原发性肿瘤中，只有一小部分肿瘤细胞发生了 EMT 过程，值得注意的是，肺转移灶主要由仍保留了上皮细胞特征的非 EMT 肿瘤细胞组成。他们进一步通过过表达 miR - 200 来抑制 EMT 过程，但这并不影响肺转移灶的形成。这个实验说明 EMT 可能并非肿瘤转移的必要条件，丰富了我们对 EMT 与肿瘤转移的认识。

三、MicroRNA 是调控上皮间充质转化的关键分子

（一） MicroRNA 的加工成熟与作用机制

miRNA 是一类由 20～24 个核苷酸构成的内源性非编码小

RNA，它们通过与 mRNA 的 3′-UTR 结合调节 60% 左右的编码基因，阻止其翻译或促进其降解。到目前为止，miRBase 数据库已收录了人体内 1870 种前体表达的 2585 条成熟 miRNA 序列。它们几乎参与到所有的生物学过程，并且在肿瘤的发生、发展中扮演着重要的角色。编码 miRNA 的基因大部分定位于基因间，也有一部分位于其他基因的内含子或外显子区。大部分 miRNA 在细胞核内由 RNA 聚合酶 Ⅱ 进行转录，经加帽、剪接、加尾生成 pri-miRNA。这些长的 pri-miRNA 经双链 RNA 酶Ⅲ Drosha 和双链 RNA 结合蛋白 DGCR8 构成的微处理器进行剪切。Drosha 含有两个 RNA 酶Ⅲ 结构域，每个 RNA 酶Ⅲ 结构域剪切 pri-miRNA 茎环结构中双链 RNA 的一条链，释放出 60~70 个核苷酸的发夹状前体 miRNA（pre-miRNA）。接着，pre-miRNA 由 exportin5 转运到细胞质，进一步被一种 RNA 酶Ⅲ Dicer1 加工成 22 个核苷酸左右的 miRNA——miRNA＊双链，并很快被引导进入 RNA 结合蛋白 TRBP 连接 Dicer1 和 Ago 蛋白组成的 miRNA 诱导的沉默复合体（miRISC），介导 miRNA 发挥生物学功能。

　　miRISC 通过 miRNA 和靶基因 mRNA 间的碱基互补配对介导基因抑制，此过程可被分为以下三类。第一类是位点特异性剪切，也称 RNA 干扰，依赖于 miRNA 与 mRNA 的完全或近完全互补配对，这一现象在哺乳动物中十分罕见。另外两类即促进 mRNA 降解和抑制翻译是哺乳动物中常见的 miRNA 作用机制。通常认为 miRNA 主要识别其靶基因 3′-UTR 的互补序列，而近期有研究报道 miRNA 也可以和 mRNA 的 5′-UTR 或开放阅读框（ORF）结合，甚至在生长抑制的条件下，miRNA 可以促进靶基因的翻译。由于 miRNA 多样灵活的作用方式，一个 miRNA 可同时调控多个 mRNA，同样一个 mRNA 亦可接受多个 miRNA 的调控。因此，miRNA 与其靶基因构成复杂的调控网络，在肿瘤的发生、发展过程中起到重要的调节作用。

（二）MicroRNA 参与 EMT 的调控

1. MicroRNA 可调控 EMT 相关的转录抑制因子

E - 钙黏素的表达减少是 EMT 过程的关键分子事件。Snail 蛋白、碱性螺旋环螺旋（bHLH）转录因子和 ZEB 蛋白是最常见的 E - 钙黏蛋白转录抑制因子。在多种肿瘤中，miRNA 可直接调控这些 EMT 转录因子。多项研究表明 miR - 200 家族和 ZEB 蛋白之间存在着重要的功能联系。miR - 200 家族由 5 个成员组成：miR - 200a/200b/429 和 miR - 200c/141。Gregory 发现 miR - 200 家族的全部成员在发生 EMT 过程的 MDCK 肾脏细胞中表达下调，相反过表达这些 miRNA 可以加强上皮细胞特性并阻断 TGFβ 诱导的 EMT 过程。而且，miR - 200 家族已被证实可通过与 ZEB1 和 ZEB2 的 3' - UTR 直接结合，转录后抑制其表达水平。有趣的是，miR - 200 家族的启动子区域含有高度保守的 ZEB 结合位点。因此，ZEB 蛋白可逆向对 miR - 200 家族发挥转录水平的控制，提示我们 miR - 200 家族和 ZEB 蛋白之间存在一个双负反馈环路。

此外，miR - 205 和 miR - 200 家族成员协同抑制 ZEB 的表达并导致 EMT 过程的逆转。在肝细胞和非小细胞肺癌中，miR - 30 均通过作用于 Snail1 抑制 TGFβ1 诱导的 EMT 过程。在肝癌细胞中 miR - 148 可负向调控 Met/Snail1 信号通路来阻断 EMT 及肿瘤转移。miR - 1 和 miR - 200 可抑制 Slug 的表达，反过来 Slug 也可转录抑制 miR - 1 和 miR - 200 的表达，形成了一个双负反馈环路，类似的负反馈环路亦发生在 miR - 34/Snail1 和 miR - 203/Snail1 之间，对 EMT 起到调控作用。这些双负反馈环路可促进 EMT 的激活并控制细胞在上皮和间充质两种状态中的平衡。近期,一个整合了 miR-203/Snail1 和 miR-200/ZEB 两个负反馈环路的 EMT 调控网络被作为控制分化及肿瘤进展过程中上皮细胞可塑性的开关而提出。

2. MicroRNA 可调控 EMT 的效应因子

miRNA 不仅可以通过调控转录因子对影响上皮或间充质表型的细胞构架组成产生间接影响,也可对其发挥直接作用。敲除 miR-155 可抑制 TGFβ 诱导的 EMT,细胞间紧密连接的解体以及肿瘤细胞的迁移与侵袭,并且这一效应是通过 miR-155 对 RhoA 的靶向抑制介导产生的。在结肠癌细胞中,经 TGFβ 处理,miR-21 和 miR-31 被诱导表达升高并促进了细胞的运动和侵袭能力,且其表达水平与淋巴结转移和远处转移呈正相关。进一步的研究表明,miR-21 和 miR-31 均通过抑制小 G 蛋白 Rac 的 GEF——TIAM1 的翻译促进 EMT 的发生。然而另有研究显示 miR-31 可通过作用于另一个靶基因 RhoA 抑制肿瘤的转移潜能。

CDH1 是 E-钙黏素的编码基因,在乳腺癌细胞中,miR-9 表达异常升高,且可以直接与 CDH1 的 3′-UTR 结合,抑制其表达来促进肿瘤细胞的迁移与侵袭能力。因为在 EMT 过程中 E-钙黏素的下调通常伴随 N-钙黏素的上调,并且在进展期胃癌细胞中,可以靶向调控 N-钙黏素的 miR-194 呈现低表达。在 TGFβ 诱导的 EMT 中,miR-491-5p 可抑制 PAR3 的表达,从而降低上皮细胞紧密连接的稳定性。

3. MicroRNA 可调控 EMT 的诱导因子

EMT 的发生、发展可由 TGFβ、Wnt、Notch 等多种信号通路来介导,miRNA 可通过调控这些信号通路中的诸多环节影响 EMT 过程。细胞因子 TGFβ 和其丝/苏氨酸激酶受体结合,激活下游的 Smad2 和 Smad3,二者和 Smad4 构成 Smad 三聚体,转位入核,转录激活 Snail、ZEB、bHLH 家族,导致上皮相关基因的抑制和间充质相关基因的活化。实际上，TGFβ 信号通路中的大多数成员均受到 miRNA 的调控。在急性髓系白血病（APL）细胞中，Zhong 发现随着全反式维甲酸的治疗，APL 细胞的分化，miR-146a 呈下降趋势，且此 miRNA 通过靶向作用于 Smad4 影响细胞的增殖能力。miR-204 可直接作用于 TGFβⅡ受体和 Slug，其表达水平降低可导致 claudin10、16、19 的下调，而 miR-204 在维持上皮完整性中有着双重角色，因为它还可以靶向于在 TGFβ 处理发生的 EMT 中迅速诱导上调的 Snail1。

在 EMT 中扮演重要角色的 miR-200 家族在此环节亦发挥着举足轻重的作用。近期 miR-200/ZEB 环路被报道与 Notch 信号通路相关联，即 Notch 信号通路相关分子 Jagged1，MAML2 和 MAML3 均是 miR-200 家族的靶基因，ZEB1 通过对 miR-200 家族的负性调控，对 Notch 通路起到激活的作用。另外有研究表明，在结肠癌细胞中，ZEB1 可受 β-catenin 直接的转录调控，并且 miR-200a 通过靶向作用于 ZEB 或 β-catenin 下调 β-catenin 介导的转录，而 miR-200b 和 miR-200c 对 β-catenin 并无明显作用。

（三）胃癌转移相关的 miRNA

一项来自 Tetsuya Ueda 等人的研究通过 353 例胃癌样本的 miRNA 芯片检测，分析得到最重要的三个与胃癌进展相关的 miRNA：miR-125b、miR-199a、miR-100。多项研究显示 miRNA 通过作用于胃癌转移级联事件中的不同要素发挥着重要的调控作用。过表达 miR-196b 可导致 E-钙黏素的下调促进胃癌转移，且 miR-200b 通过靶向作用于 ZEB2 抑制胃癌转移。上调 miR-27 可增加 EMT 相关基因的表达，包括 ZEB1、ZEB2、Slug、Vimentin 并降低 E-钙黏素的表达。除了 E-钙黏素和它的调控因子外，细胞外基质重塑蛋白和细胞黏附分子亦受miRNA的控制。胃癌细胞中 miR - 21 的上调可促进细胞的迁移和侵袭能力，其主要通过 miR - 21 介导的 MMP 的抑制剂 RECK的下调而实现。miR - 10b 在淋巴结转移阳性的胃癌组织中的表达较无转移胃癌组织中显著上调，这一作用通过抑制其靶基因HOXD10 激活 RhoC 和 AKT 所介导。ROCK1 可促进多种类型肿瘤的侵袭转移，而胃癌中 miR - 148a 可直接和 ROCK1 的 3′ -UTR 区结合，降低其表达从而抑制肿瘤转移。此外，miR - 145通过靶基因 N - 钙黏素和 MMP9；miR - 429 通过靶基因 Myc，miR - 409 通过靶基因 RDX，一个肿瘤转移促进分子；miR - 335通过靶基因 BCLW 和 SP1，均发挥抗胃癌转移作用。

随着 miRNA 研究的快速进展，本实验室也很快认识到 miRNA作为重要的调控分子在肿瘤发生、发展的各个阶段起到重要作用，并在此领域进行了一系列功能和机制的研究。我们利用miRNA 芯片结合本实验室自主构建的高低转移细胞系 MKN28M/NM 及 SGC7901M/NM 筛选差异表达的 miRNA，得到在两株高转移细胞系中 11 个上调和 34 个下调的 miRNA，miR - 218 是其中一个显著下调的 miRNA，进一步我们证实 miR - 218 在胃癌中表达降低，miR - 218 作为 Slit3 基因的内含子 miRNA，与其宿主基因一同转录，当 Slit3/miR - 218 表达下调时，miR - 218 的靶基因 Robo1 表达水平升高，进而与其配体 Slit2 相互作用促进胃癌转移。通过对另一对高低转移细胞系 GC9811 - P 和 GC9811 进行高通量的 miRNA 表达谱检测，我们对其中差异表达的 miR - 7和 let - 7f 进行了深入研究。体内外实验均证明 miR - 7 可抑制胃癌细胞的侵袭转移能力，其主要作用机制是通过靶向调控胰岛素生长因子受体（IGF1R）导致 Snail 下调从而抑制 EMT 的发生。我们还发现 let - 7f 通过抑制靶基因非肌肉肌球蛋白重链 ⅡA（MYH9）的表达，发挥胃癌细胞迁移和侵袭的抑制作用。血清反应因子 SRF 可与 miR－199a 的启动子结合，转录激活并上调 miR－199a－5p 及 miR－199a－3p 的表达，上调的 miR－199a－5p 可介导 E－钙黏素的下降推动 EMT 过程的发生从而促进胃癌细胞转移。此外，我们鉴定出表观遗传学调控因子 UHRF1 受 miR－146a/b 的直接调控表达下调，使其下游 Slit3、CDH4、RUNX3 抑癌基因启动子去甲基化而重新激活，进而抑制转移的发生。

四、miR－2392 在胃癌转移中的作用和机制

本实验室前期研究发现甲基化调节因子 UHRF1 在胃癌中表达明显升高，可促进胃癌细胞的体内外增殖和体内外侵袭转移，于胃癌发生、发展过程中发挥重要作用。由于 UHRF1 作为一种表观遗传学调控分子，可在转录水平调控基因表达。因此，为探索 UHRF1 能否通过调控 miRNA 来发挥功能，我们通过对 UHRF1 下游 miRNA 芯片进行生物信息学分析及候选 miRNA 的表达检测，筛选到受 UHRF1 调控的 miR－2392。经 qRT－PCR 和原位杂交检测，miR－2392 在胃癌细胞和组织中的表达显著高于相应的癌旁组织和永生化胃上皮细胞。同时，miR－2392 的表达与患者的 TNM 分期和生存时间密切相关，miR－2392 表达越低，患者的分期越高、生存时间越短，提示 miR－2392 可作为病情与预后评估的分子标志物。

随后的体内外功能获得和缺失实验证实 miR－2392 可调节胃癌细胞的迁移与侵袭能力。通过生物信息学分析筛选到 miR－2392 的候选靶基因。通过 Western Blot、qRT－PCR 和双荧光素酶报告基因实验证明了 MAML3 和 WHSC1 是 miR－2392 的直接靶基因。对 MAML3 和 WHSC1 进行体外功能实验及补救实验进

一步验证了 miR－2392 通过作用于 MAML3 和 WHSC1 而影响胃癌细胞的迁移与侵袭。

我们观察到，胃癌细胞过表达 miR－2392 后，细胞形态由梭形转变为组织相对紧密的圆形或鹅卵石，并且通过 EMT 标志物的检测，我们证实了 miR－2392 可抑制 EMT 的发生。这一过程一方面通过下调 MAML3－Notch 的转录共激活因子，导致 Notch 通路活性降低，下游 Slug、Twist1 表达减少；另一方面通过下调 WHSC1 减弱了 Twist1 的表达。此外 WHSC1 既受 miR－2392 的负向调控亦受 MAML3 的正向调控，且 MAML3 对 Twist1 的影响是通过调控 WHSC1 引发的间接作用。

最后，经免疫组织化学检测，与 miR－2392 表达模式相反，MAML3 和 WHSC1 在胃组织中的表达显著高于相应的癌旁组织，且与患者的 TNM 分期和生存时间密切相关，MAML3 和 WHSC1 表达越高，患者的分期越高、生存时间越短。相关性分析证实 miR－2392 与 MAML3、WHSC1 在组织中的表达呈负相关，为 miR－2392－MAML3/WHSC1 的调控关系提供了临床证据。

（李进晶）

参考文献

[1] Torre LA, Bray F, Siegel RL, et al. Global cancer statistics, 2012. CA Cancer J Clin, 2015, 65: 87 – 108.

[2] Chen W, Zheng R, Baade PD, et al. Cancer statistics in China, 2015. CA Cancer J Clin, 2016, 66: 115 – 132.

[3] Gupta GP, Massague J. Cancer metastasis: building a framework. Cell, 2006, 127: 679 – 695.

[4] Chaffer CL, Weinberg RA. A perspective on cancer cell metastasis. Science, 2011, 331: 1559 – 1564.

[5] Escribese MM, Casas M, Corbi AL. Influence of low oxygen tensions on macrophage polarization. Immunobiology, 2012, 217: 1233 – 1240.

[6] Mantovani A, Sica A. Macrophages, innate immunity and cancer: balance, tolerance, and diversity. Curr Opin Immunol, 2010, 22: 231 – 237.

[7] Gocheva V, Wang HW, Gadea BB, et al. IL – 4 induces cathepsin protease activity in tumor – associated macrophages to promote cancer growth and invasion. Genes Dev, 2010, 24: 241 – 255.

[8] Qian BZ, Pollard JW. Macrophage diversity enhances tumor progression and metastasis. Cell, 2010, 141: 39 – 51.

[9] Sidani M, Wyckoff J, Xue C, et al. Probing the microenvironment of mammary tumors using multiphoton microscopy. J Mammary Gland Biol Neoplasia, 2006, 11: 151 – 163.

[10] Talmadge JE, Gabrilovich DI. History of myeloid – derived suppressor cells. Nat Rev Cancer, 2013, 13: 739 – 752.

[11] Diaz – Montero CM, Salem ML, Nishimura MI, et al. Increased circulating myeloid – derived suppressor cells correlate with clinical cancer stage, metastatic tumor burden, and doxorubicin – cyclophosphamide chemotherapy. Cancer Immunol Immunother, 2009, 58: 49 – 59.

[12] Shirota Y, Shirota H, Klinman DM. Intratumoral injection of CpG oligonucleotides induces the differentiation and reduces the immunosuppressive activity of myeloid – derived suppressor cells. J Immunol, 2012, 188: 1592 – 1599.

[13] Sceneay J, Smyth MJ, Moller A. The pre – metastatic niche: finding common ground. Cancer Metastasis Rev, 2013, 32: 449 – 464.

[14] Erler JT, Bennewith KL, Nicolau M, et al. Lysyl oxidase is essential for hypoxia – induced metastasis. Nature, 2006, 440: 1222 – 1226.

[15] Sceneay J, Chow MT, Chen A, et al. Primary tumor hypoxia recruits CD11b + /Ly6Cmed/Ly6G + immune suppressor cells and compromises NK cell cytotoxicity in the premetastatic niche. Cancer Res, 2012, 72: 3906 – 3911.

[16] Psaila B, Lyden D. The metastatic niche: adapting the foreign soil. Nat

Rev Cancer, 2009, 9: 285 – 293.

[17] Peinado H, Aleckovic M, Lavotshkin S, et al. Melanoma exosomes educate bone marrow progenitor cells toward a pro – metastatic phenotype through MET. Nat Med, 2012, 18: 883 – 891.

[18] Thiery JP, Acloque H, Huang RY, et al. Epithelial – mesenchymal transitions in development and disease. Cell, 2009, 139: 871 – 890.

[19] Ohtani S, Terashima M, Satoh J, et al. Expression of tight – junction – associated proteins in human gastric cancer: downregulation of claudin – 4 correlates with tumor aggressiveness and survival. Gastric Cancer, 2009, 12: 43 – 51.

[20] Niehrs C. The complex world of WNT receptor signalling. Nat Rev Mol Cell Biol, 2012, 13: 767 – 779.

[21] Kourtidis A, Ngok SP, Anastasiadis PZ. p120 catenin: an essential regulator of cadherin stability, adhesion – induced signaling, and cancer progression. Prog Mol Biol Transl Sci, 2013, 116: 409 – 432.

[22] Hoot KE, Lighthall J, Han G, et al. Keratinocyte – specific Smad2 ablation results in increased epithelial – mesenchymal transition during skin cancer formation and progression. J Clin Invest, 2008, 118: 2722 – 2732.

[23] Morita T, Mayanagi T, Sobue K. Dual roles of myocardin – related transcription factors in epithelial mesenchymal transition via slug induction and actin remodeling. J Cell Biol, 2007, 179: 1027 – 1042.

[24] Lo HW, Hsu SC, Xia W, et al. Epidermal growth factor receptor cooperates with signal transducer and activator of transcription 3 to induce epithelial – mesenchymal transition in cancer cells via up – regulation of TWIST gene expression. Cancer Res, 2007, 67: 9066 – 9076.

[25] Xie M, Zhang L, He CS, et al. Activation of Notch – 1 enhances epithelial – mesenchymal transition in gefitinib – acquired resistant lung cancer cells. J Cell Biochem, 2012, 113: 1501 – 1513.

[26] Theveneau E, Mayor R. Cadherins in collective cell migration of mesenchymal cells. Curr Opin Cell Biol, 2012, 24: 677 – 684.

[27] Brieher WM, Yap AS. Cadherin junctions and their cytoskeleton(s). Curr

Opin Cell Biol, 2013, 25: 39 –46.

[28] Hansen SM, Berezin V, Bock E. Signaling mechanisms of neurite out-growth induced by the cell adhesion molecules NCAM and N – cadherin. Cell Mol Life Sci, 2008, 65: 3809 –3821.

[29] St Johnston D, Ahringer J. Cell polarity in eggs and epithelia: parallels and diversity. Cell, 2010, 141: 757 –774.

[30] Moreno – Bueno G, Portillo F, Cano A. Transcriptional regulation of cell polarity in EMT and cancer. Oncogene, 2008, 27: 6958 –6969.

[31] Yang X, Pursell B, Lu S, et al. Regulation of beta 4 – integrin expression by epigenetic modifications in the mammary gland and during the epithelial –to –mesenchymal transition. J Cell Sci, 2009, 122:2473 –2480.

[32] Kessenbrock K, Plaks V, Werb Z. Matrix metalloproteinases: regulators of the tumor microenvironment. Cell, 2010, 141: 52 –67.

[33] Cai J, Li R, Xu X, et al. URGCP promotes non – small cell lung cancer invasiveness by activating the NF – kappaB – MMP – 9 pathway. Oncotar-get, 2015, 6: 36489 –36504.

[34] Lu YC, Chang JT, Liao CT, et al. OncomiR – 196 promotes an invasive phenotype in oral cancer through the NME4 – JNK – TIMP1 – MMP signa-ling pathway. Mol Cancer, 2014, 13: 218.

[35] Matsuoka T, Yashiro M. Rho/ROCK signaling in motility and metastasis of gastric cancer. World J Gastroenterol, 2014, 20: 13756 –13766.

[36] Fischer KR, Durrans A, Lee S, et al. Epithelial – to – mesenchymal tran-sition is not required for lung metastasis but contributes to chemoresis-tance. Nature, 2015, 527: 472 –476.

[37] Park SM, Gaur AB, Lengyel E, et al. The miR – 200 family determines the epithelial phenotype of cancer cells by targeting the E – cadherin re-pressors ZEB1 and ZEB2. Genes Dev, 2008, 22: 894 –907.

[38] Iorio MV, Croce CM. MicroRNA dysregulation in cancer: diagnostics, monitoring and therapeutics. A comprehensive review. EMBO Mol Med, 2012, 4: 143 –159.

[39] Moretti F, Thermann R, Hentze MW. Mechanism of translational regula-

tion by miR – 2 from sites in the 5′untranslated region or the open reading frame. Rna, 2010, 16: 2493 – 2502.

[40] Vasudevan S, Tong Y, Steitz JA. Switching from repression to activation: microRNAs can up – regulate translation. Science, 2007, 318: 1931 – 1934.

[41] Korpal M, Lee ES, Hu G, et al. The miR – 200 family inhibits epithelial – mesenchymal transition and cancer cell migration by direct targeting of E – cadherin transcriptional repressors ZEB1 and ZEB2. J Biol Chem, 2008, 283: 14910 – 14914.

[42] Gregory PA, Bert AG, Paterson EL, et al. The miR – 200 family and miR – 205 regulate epithelial to mesenchymal transition by targeting ZEB1 and SIP1. Nat Cell Biol, 2008, 10: 593 – 601.

[43] Bracken CP, Gregory PA, Kolesnikoff N, et al. A double – negative feedback loop between ZEB1 – SIP1 and the microRNA – 200 family regulates epithelial – mesenchymal transition. Cancer Res, 2008, 68: 7846 – 7854.

[44] Zhang J, Zhang H, Liu J, et al. miR – 30 inhibits TGF – beta1 – induced epithelial – to – mesenchymal transition in hepatocyte by targeting Snail1. Biochem Biophys Res Commun, 2012, 417: 1100 – 1105.

[45] Kumarswamy R, Mudduluru G, Ceppi P, et al. MicroRNA – 30a inhibits epithelial – to – mesenchymal transition by targeting Snail and is downregulated in non – small cell lung cancer. Int J Cancer, 2012, 130: 2044 – 2053.

[46] Zhang JP, Zeng C, Xu L, et al. MicroRNA – 148a suppresses the epithelial – mesenchymal transition and metastasis of hepatoma cells by targeting Met/Snail signaling. Oncogene, 2014, 33: 4069 – 4076.

[47] Liu YN, Yin JJ, Abou – Kheir W, et al. MiR – 1 and miR – 200 inhibit EMT via Slug – dependent and tumorigenesis via Slug – independent mechanisms. Oncogene, 2013, 32: 296 – 306.

[48] Siemens H, Jackstadt R, Hunten S, et al. miR – 34 and SNAIL form a double – negative feedback loop to regulate epithelial – mesenchymal transitions. Cell Cycle, 2011, 10: 4256 – 4271.

[49] Moes M, Le Bechec A, Crespo I, et al. A novel network integrating a miRNA – 203/SNAI1 feedback loop which regulates epithelial to mesen-

chymal transition. PLoS One, 2012, 7: e35440.

[50] Kong W, Yang H, He L, et al. MicroRNA – 155 is regulated by the trans-forming growth factor beta/Smad pathway and contributes to epithelial cell plasticity by targeting RhoA. Mol Cell Biol, 2008, 28: 6773 – 6784.

[51] Slaby O, Svoboda M, Fabian P, et al. Altered expression of miR – 21, miR – 31, miR – 143 and miR – 145 is related to clinicopathologic fea-tures of colorectal cancer. Oncology, 2007, 72: 397 – 402.

[52] Cottonham CL, Kaneko S, Xu L. miR – 21 and miR – 31 converge on TI-AM1 to regulate migration and invasion of colon carcinoma cells. J Biol Chem, 2010, 285: 35293 – 35302.

[53] Valastyan S, Chang A, Benaich N, et al. Activation of miR – 31 function in already – established metastases elicits metastatic regression. Genes Dev, 2011, 25: 646 – 659.

[54] Ma L, Young J, Prabhala H, et al. miR – 9, a MYC/MYCN – activated microRNA, regulates E – cadherin and cancer metastasis. Nat Cell Biol, 2010, 12: 247 – 256.

[55] Song Y, Zhao F, Wang Z, et al. Inverse association between miR – 194 expression and tumor invasion in gastric cancer. Ann Surg Oncol, 2012, 19: S509 – 517.

[56] Zhou Q, Fan J, Ding X, et al. TGF – beta – induced MiR – 491 – 5p ex-pression promotes Par – 3 degradation in rat proximal tubular epithelial cells. J Biol Chem, 2010, 285: 40019 – 40027.

[57] Zhong H, Wang HR, Yang S, et al. Targeting Smad4 links microRNA – 146a to the TGF – beta pathway during retinoid acid induction in acute promyelocytic leukemia cell line. Int J Hematol, 2010, 92: 129 – 135.

[58] Wang FE, Zhang C, Maminishkis A, et al. MicroRNA – 204/211 alters epithelial physiology. Faseb J, 2010, 24: 1552 – 1571.

[59] Brabletz S, Bajdak K, Meidhof S, et al. The ZEB1/miR – 200 feedback loop controls Notch signalling in cancer cells. EMBO J, 2011, 30: 770 – 782.

[60] Ueda T, Volinia S, Okumura H, et al. Relation between microRNA ex-

pression and progression and prognosis of gastric cancer: a microRNA expression analysis. Lancet Oncol, 2010, 11: 136 – 146.

[61] Liao YL, Hu LY, Tsai KW, et al. Transcriptional regulation of miR – 196b by ETS2 in gastric cancer cells. Carcinogenesis, 2012, 33: 760 – 769.

[62] Kurashige J, Kamohara H, Watanabe M, et al. MicroRNA – 200b regulates cell proliferation, invasion, and migration by directly targeting ZEB2 in gastric carcinoma. Ann Surg Oncol, 2012, 19: S656 – 664.

[63] Zhang Z, Liu S, Shi R, et al. miR – 27 promotes human gastric cancer cell metastasis by inducing epithelial – to – mesenchymal transition. Cancer Genet, 2011, 204: 486 – 491.

[64] Zhang Z, Li Z, Gao C, et al. miR – 21 plays a pivotal role in gastric cancer pathogenesis and progression. Lab Invest, 2008, 88: 1358 – 1366.

[65] Liu Z, Zhu J, Cao H, et al. miR – 10b promotes cell invasion through RhoC – AKT signaling pathway by targeting HOXD10 in gastric cancer. Int J Oncol, 2012, 40: 1553 – 1560.

[66] Zheng B, Liang L, Wang C, et al. MicroRNA – 148a suppresses tumor cell invasion and metastasis by downregulating ROCK1 in gastric cancer. Clin Cancer Res, 2011, 17: 7574 – 7583.

[67] Gao P, Xing AY, Zhou GY, et al. The molecular mechanism of microRNA – 145 to suppress invasion – metastasis cascade in gastric cancer. Oncogene, 2013, 32: 491 – 501.

[68] Sun T, Wang C, Xing J, et al. miR – 429 modulates the expression of c – myc in human gastric carcinoma cells. Eur J Cancer, 2011, 47: 2552 – 2559.

[69] Zheng B, Liang L, Huang S, et al. MicroRNA – 409 suppresses tumour cell invasion and metastasis by directly targeting radixin in gastric cancers. Oncogene, 2012, 31: 4509 – 4516.

[70] Xu Y, Zhao F, Wang Z, et al. MicroRNA – 335 acts as a metastasis suppressor in gastric cancer by targeting Bcl – w and specificity protein 1. Oncogene, 2012, 31: 1398 – 1407.

[71] Tie J, Pan Y, Zhao L, et al. MiR – 218 inhibits invasion and metastasis

of gastric cancer by targeting the Robo1 receptor. PLoS Genet, 2010, 6: e1000879.

[72] Zhao X, Dou W, He L, et al. MicroRNA − 7 functions as an anti − metastatic microRNA in gastric cancer by targeting insulin − like growth factor − 1 receptor. Oncogene, 2013, 32: 1363 − 1372.

[73] Liang S, He L, Zhao X, et al. MicroRNA let − 7f inhibits tumor invasion and metastasis by targeting MYH9 in human gastric cancer. PLoS One, 2011, 6: e18409.

[74] Zhao X, He L, Li T, et al. SRF expedites metastasis and modulates the epithelial to mesenchymal transition by regulating miR − 199a − 5p expression in human gastric cancer. Cell Death Differ, 2014, 21: 1900 − 1913.

[75] Zhou L, Zhao X, Han Y, et al. Regulation of UHRF1 by miR − 146a/b modulates gastric cancer invasion and metastasis. Faseb J, 2013, 27: 4929 − 4939.

第六章

环状 RNAs 分子的形成、特征及潜在临床应用

自人们第一次通过电子显微镜发现环形 RNA 的存在迄今已 30 余年,早在 1989 年,T. O. Diener 提出植物中的环状 RNA (circRNAs)因其体积小且为环状的特点能够在易于出错的原始 RNA 自我复制系统中存活,并在不需要初始及终止信号的前提下保证了完全复制,因此,这种环状 RNA 相较内含子而言更有可能是前细胞 RNA 界的"活化石"。并且,长期以来,环状 RNA 被认为是一种来源于异常 RNA 剪接或某些病原体如 δ 型肝炎病毒及某些植物病毒的产物的"分子意外事件"。直到近年来,人们发现大量环状 RNA 分子不仅是为哺乳动物细胞内源性 RNA,在细胞中含量丰富、结构稳定,而且外显子环状 RNA 及内含子环状 RNA 都具备调节基因表达的潜在功能。

一、环状 RNA 分子形成机制及其调节

人类第一次发现内源性环状 RNA 是在 20 世纪 90 年代初期研究人类细胞 DCC 转录本时。当时,该研究的研究者描述了一类具有异于常规顺序排列的外显子的转录本,即 5′外显子被"拖曳"至 3′外显子下游,而且,尽管如此,这些外显子仍然保持了完整性并且使用了常规的剪接供体及受体位点。这种排布方式被称作"外显子拖曳"。这些发生"外显子拖曳"的转录本比预期的转录

本少了几个数量级且没有多聚腺苷酸尾,主要表达于细胞质,并在人及大鼠组织中均有表达。该研究者推测该类产物可能从分子内剪接生成进而产生外显子环状 RNA。该基因一预期下游外显子 3′尾位点被连接在另一正常情况下应位于上游的外显子 5′头端部位,这种剪接方式称为"后剪接"。

之后,又有其他研究报道了在人、小鼠及大鼠细胞中"拖曳转录本"的存在,如 ETS – 1、Sry12 及 CYP Ⅱ C24 等。这些研究都是偶然间在分析 PCR 产物时发现了"后剪接"转录本的存在。Sry 通常不发生剪接,但其经典剪接位点 GT/AG 序列却与"后剪接"有关,提示经典剪接体或参与"后剪接"过程(图 6 – 1),Starke 等的研究亦证实经典剪接信号对于外显子环状 RNA 分子形成的必要性(图 6 – 2)。并且,ETS – 1 及 CYPIIC24 外显子环状 RNA 应用的剪接供体及受体剪接点也涉及"前剪接"过程。在随后二十余年又发现数个环状 RNA,但它们在细胞中的丰度通常远远小于源基因所产生的线性产物。Steven Kelly 等的研究还发现,外显子环化不仅普遍,并且常与外显子跳跃有关,这一特征又显著增加了人类转录本调控机制的复杂性。

据报道,哺乳动物外显子环状 RNA 的形成机制大致有两种,都涉及经典剪接子导致的后剪接过程。第一个机制即"直接后剪接"(曾被称为"误剪接"),是一下游剪接供体与以未剪接的上游剪接受体相配对;第二个机制即"套索中间体"或"外显子跳跃"机制,是外显子跳跃所产生的套索间相剪接连接。并且,前者发生率要显著高于后者(图 6 – 3)。

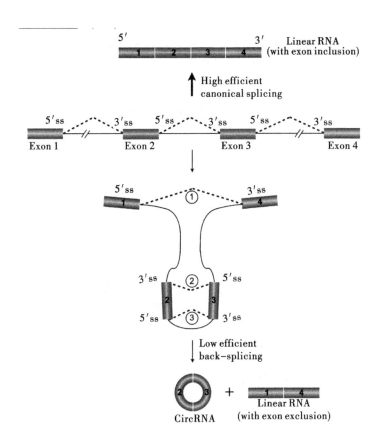

图 6 − 1　后剪接机制示意图

（引自 RNA Biol,2015,12:381 − 388）

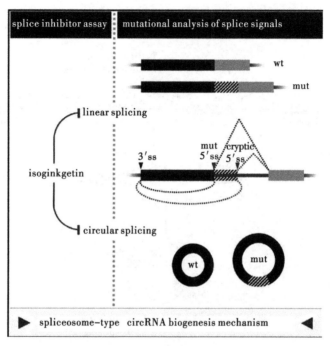

图 6 - 2　经典剪接信号在外显子环状 RNA 分子形成过程的重要作用

（引自 Cell Rep,2015,10:103 - 111）

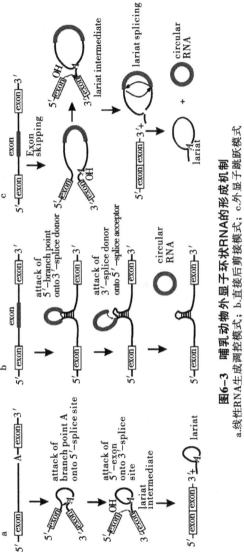

图6-3 哺乳动物外显子环状RNA的形成机制

a.线性RNA生成调控模式；b.直接后剪接模式；c.外显子跳跃模式
（引自Nucleic Acids Res, 2015, 43: 2454-2465）

　　此外,Simon J. Conn 等发现在人细胞发生上皮 – 间充质转化
过程中有成百上千的环状 RNA 分子被调节,并且超过 1/3 以上的
环状 RNA 分子被可替代剪接因子 quaking(QKI)所调节,通过改
变 QKI 的水平,环状 RNA 分子丰度亦依赖于内含子 QKI 结合基
序而不同(图 6 – 4)。

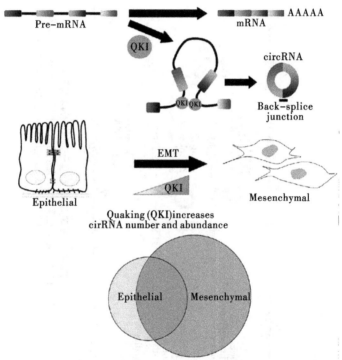

图 6 – 4　可替代剪接因子 quaking(QKI)调节环状 RNA 分子生成机制
(引自 Cell,2015,160:1125 – 1134)

二、环状 RNA 分子的检测方法

在大规模并行测序时代到来前,环状 RNA 的重要性远未阐释清楚。大多数环状 RNA 直到近来才得以鉴定的原因有以下几点:首先,与 miRNAs 及其他小 RNAs 不同,circRNAs 不容易通过体积法或电泳迁移法从其他 RNA 分子中分离出来。常规分子技术要求进行扩增或者/以及循环碎片破碎,由于 circRNAs 没有游离的 3′或 5′端,因此就无法通过依靠游离多聚腺苷酸尾〔如 cDNA 末端快速扩增法、poly(A) 富集 RNA – 测序法等〕的分子技术对其进行分离鉴别。而且,circRNAs 的一个关键特征即:被称为"后剪接"的外显子无序排布也非环状 RNA 所独有,并且早期 RNA 测序绘图算法也过滤掉了类似序列。这些问题都通过外显子核酸酶为基础的富集方法、新的生物信息学工具、高通量长读取测序以及对去除核糖体 RNA 的 RNA 数据库(而非 polyA 富集的数据库)进行测序等得以解决。目前,环状 RNA 的检测方法主要有几下几种:

(一)鉴别后剪接

基于测序为基础的方法使人们对环状 RNA 有了更多的认识,发现与后剪接构造一致的序列是证实外显子环状 RNA 生成的关键证据。这里,将具有与释模板相反外显子排序的序列称为"显后剪接",尤其是,显后剪接序列或许是通过不同于外显子环状 RNA 形成的其他机制而生成,譬如逆转录酶模板转换、串联重复及 RNA 反式剪接等(图 6 – 5A:形成显后剪接的几种机制,本示意图中,长方形代表外显子,横线代表内含子,转录方向用右向箭头表示,直角折线表示常规剪接,弧形表示后剪接。①逆转录酶模板转换,在此过程中,逆转录酶转录了其上游外显子的另一份拷贝;②DNA模板的串联重复导致重复外显子生成;③反后剪接即一RNA分子被剪接至另一RNA分子上;④外显子环状RNA可通过顺式-后剪接将来源于同一RNA分子的外显子剪接在一起形成环状)。

　　逆转录酶模板转换是一cDNA合成产物,其常常以同源依赖性方式在一延伸DNA分子从其模板RNA分子解离下来及从另一RNA模板恢复延伸时产生。这就造成一种后剪接产物的假象,容易对分析稀有剪接产物造成干扰。然而,大部分模板转换均是随机发生并且不会产生大量的具有同一序列的cDNA分子。因此,若某一cDNA数据库中的显后剪接序列为高丰度的话就证明其也在RNA模板表达。这可以用鉴别多独特读取深度测序或"相向"qPCR引物进行评估。当后剪接事件将外在序列剪接在一起时,这些"相向"引物在基因扩增时彼此向相反方向但最终"融合"并扩增成一非连续性扩增子(图6-5B-i)。或者,后剪接序列在RNA池中的出现也可直接用RNA酶保护法或者northern blot探针检测后剪接序列法进行评估(图6-5B-ii-vi)(图6-5B:区分环状RNA与其他后剪接产物的分子生物学方法示意图。i,一对相向引物各自向外延伸产物形成扩增子,通过后剪接相结合;ii,经典线状RNA、外显子环状RNA及由反式剪接或串联复制而来RNA在变性琼脂糖凝胶中的相对迁移距离;iii,经过RNase H处理后的RNA琼脂糖凝胶电泳图,只有环状RNA仍为一条单一条带;iv,通过两种不同交联聚丙烯酰凝胶进行2D凝胶电泳可见环状RNA呈一非对角曲线;v,凝胶捕获实验可将环状RNA滞留于电泳槽孔中,而线形RNA则可进行迁移)。

　　显后剪接序列也可由串联DNA复制而来,后者可在一个基因内产生复制的外显子。当这些序列被转录时,mRNA就因注释模板序列与细胞内DNA模板之间的不同而包含一显后剪接序列(图6-5A-ii)。而且,当反式剪接(一种两个不同分子参与剪接的过程)发生于两个同一基因形成的 RNA 分子间时也能产生显后剪接子(图 6 - 5A - iii)。有几种区分真外显子环状 RNA 与这些产物的方法(图 6 - 5A - iv)。线形 RNA 常有 3′多聚腺苷酸尾,而环状 RNA 没有。在凝胶电泳中,外显子环状 RNA 较线形 RNA 分子迁移慢(图 6 - 5B)。然而,外显子环状 RNA 比来自同一基因的全长、反式剪接的或串联重复的转录本的核苷酸序列少,因此较少发生交联,在凝胶种迁移速度也较快(图 6 - 5B - ii)。此外,也可用标准的 northern blot 实验分析这一特质。通过弱水解作用或靶向 RNase H 降解可更加明确这一结果。经 RNase H 降解或水解出一处断端后,环状 RNA 可呈一线状产物(图 6 - 5B - iii),2D 凝胶电泳及凝胶捕获实验更加证实了这一点(图 6 - 5B - iv - v)。在 2D 凝胶电泳中,环状 RNA 在高度交联凝胶中比低度交联凝胶中的迁移能力弱。在凝胶捕获实验中,环状 RNA 与融化的琼脂糖凝胶融合交联被捕获,因此在外加电场中就不再迁移。酶解法也可证实环状 RNA 的存在。RNase R 核酸外切酶,烟草酸性磷酸酶及终止子核酸外切酶都无法酶解环状 RNA 但却可以有效降解大多数线形 RNA 分子。在所有这些情况中,在处理前后对 RNA 分子进行的量化分析显示环状 RNA 转录本具有一定的丰度。最后,应用足够长序列读取或配对末端读取法,就可能鉴别出与环状 RNA 不同的序列。这些可能即含有显后剪接序列也含有后剪接拟物外的外显子序列。譬如,一来源于更长的包含外显子 4 和 5 的序列中的外显子 3 及 2 构成的显后剪接能最好地被反式剪接 RNA 理论解释。上述所有方法都有其局限性,将其结合起来能够更好的鉴定环状 RNA。

将环状 RNA 与套索 RNA 分子区分开来非常重要。套索 RNA 是在经典 RNA 分子剪接过程中形成,且许多套索 RNA 由高表达、非多聚腺苷酸尾的内含子序列构成,并在剪接分支点处有 2′—5′碳连接,其结构往往比预期的更加稳定。这些稳定的套索 RNA3′尾端降解后留下残端分子,这样的套索产物曾被称为"环状内含子 RNA",因其具有 2′—5′连接,因而可与外显子环状 RNA 相区分。外显子环状 RNA 没有 2′—5′连接,但在整个分子中都具有 3′—5′连接。

如上所述,套索 RNA 与外显子环状 RNA 在外形上有相似之处。它们通常都对核酸外切酶敏感,比线形 RNA 迁移偏慢,当在环的某处出现一缺口时也形成一单一条带。然而,外显子环状 RNA 因其显后剪接序列特征容易与内含子环状 RNA、套索 RNA 等相区分开来。在套索 RNA 的分支点处,也可有低效率地逆转录现象,产生一表面上与后剪接类似的序列,即具有并列的上下游序列。但是,这些分支点逆转录序列含有内含子序列,尤其是经典剪接供体位点以及分支点核苷酸 5′ GT。而且,当逆转录酶跨过 2′—5′连接时,会产生一个或更多的非模板碱基,这些碱基可通过测序辨认识别。这一特征可用于为内含子产物排除外显子环状 RNA 起源的产物。原则上,因核酸外切酶选择性地水解 2′—5′连接,通过脱支酶处理后再用该酶消化,可优先将套索 RNA 从其他环状产物排除掉。因此,尽管套索是常见的环状 RNA 分子,也能将其容易地与外显子环状 RNA 区分开来。

(二)基因组方法

由于测序技术(深度长读取测序)的发展、RNA 基因源性定位算法优化以及核糖体 RNA 去除策略(可实现非多聚核苷酸尾RNA 测序)的使用使得环状 RNA 全基因组分析成为可能。总体来说,可以采取两种方法:①从现存在的转录样本中获取待选连接;②应用剪接比对算法将读取与基因组序列比对。这两种方法都鉴定出了可被测序法、RNase R 核酸外切酶实验检测及其他方法证实的环状 RNA。第一个通过基因组学方法鉴定出的外显子环状 RNA 是意外地在一 cDNA 片段配对末端读取独立定位过程中发现的。这种方法鉴定出了大量从未预料到的片段存在,这些片段中两读取对定位于同一基因但却与预期的基因注释方向相反(图 6 – 5Ca)(图 6 – 5Ca:当读取对在一个或更多剪接位点具有相反方向时,配对末端读取可定位于注释的转录本以及推测的后剪接位置)。意识到这些片段可能来源于环状 RNA,人们又用已有的基因注释把后剪接的定位进行估算。该法又通过在固定窗内叠瓦式无序配对末端读取扫描得以扩展(图 6 – 5Cb)(图 6 – 5Cb:配对末端读取可直接定位于基因组,大量读取定位超出基因顺序提示附近或许有后剪接存在,尤其是当大量读取聚集于基因组设定叠瓦长度的固定"窗")。这个策略具有分析快速分子 rRNA 去除数据库中的优势,但主要是基于候选策略即依赖于从已有基因中构建的环状 RNA,因此并不能从未注释转录本中检测出环状 RNA 也不能提供环状的直接证据。然而,对大量个别物种的 qPCR 实验显示转录本基本上都抵抗 RNase R 核酸外切酶作用并缺乏包含线形 RNA 分子(反式剪接或复制产物)的后剪接所预期的特征。其他应用 rRNA – 删除库的方法包括从哺乳动物细胞及线虫细胞 rRNA – 删除 RNA 序列数据库中鉴别具有显后剪接的读取,而非基于候选策略的方法,即将读取在基因组位置上重新进行定位并在每个读取中鉴定出显后剪接序列。他们选择了不能直接定位于基因组的读取然后将每一读取两端分别定位,这样就可以在单核苷酸水平上鉴定出推测的后剪接,并鉴定出未注释的剪接位点,不过这种方法可能不如候选策略法敏感(图 6 – 5Cc)(图 6 – 5Cc:一个读取可以被分割成几个片段,因此一个读取的几个部分可以被定位于基因组的不同部位,通过这种方法可以在核苷酸水平在没有既定注释前体下定位后剪接)。

此外,一个更微妙的基于候选策略的分析方法即不用核酸外切酶富集的 rRNA – 删除 RNA 测序法。此方法应用深度测序及 75 – bp 末端配对读取鉴定定位于以现有基因注释获得的候选连接处的显后剪接序列。在该法中,将读取对分开,每一个读取都包含一个显后剪接,该显后剪接有两种,一种是没有定位于后剪接外显子之间外显子的后剪接读取,因此其可能源于环状 RNA(图 6 –5Da:与潜在外显子环状 RNA 不一致的配对末端。例 1,读取对的第一个读取定位于后剪接,但其配对读取因位于一不涉及后剪接的外显子,不符合环状 RNA;例 2,读取对的第一个读取定位于后剪接,但该读取对定位于一涉及后剪接的外显子之间的外显子,符合环状RNA);另一种是读取对中的第二个读取定位于一后剪接外显子外的外显子,因此就不能用环状 RNA 来解释。人们推测第二种或许是一种测序"赝品"。两组的定位质量统计学分布都被用于为每一个观察到的连接产生信度评分(图 6 –5Db:应用两对读取获取两个分布,该分布可用于设置基于定位质量特征的经验错误发生率),并且,这种方法可使用错误发现概率终止法而不是随机深度读取法。除了基于测序的方法外,还有一种被称为"环状测序"的用于全基因组环状 RNA 鉴定的生物信息学方法,即在高通量测序前先应用 RNase R 消化以此鉴别不被其消化的序列片段(图 6 –5Ea)。

　　该方法应用能够鉴定显后剪接序列的定位算式而非需要外显子顺序的算式。在哺乳动物而非古生菌中,需要将 rRNA 去除掉。应用该方法,就可能在两个特征上鉴定出外显子环状 RNA:①应用片段定位法可鉴定出包含后剪接的读取(图 6 – 5Eb);②与模拟组相比,从环状产物而来的读取可显著富集于 RNase R 处理后的样品中(通常为 8 ~16 倍)。应通过核酸外切酶去除线形 RNA 外显子,同样,环状 RNA 中也不应出现剪接连接。

　　环状测序亦可鉴定套索 RNA 分子,如前所述,套索 RNA 分子在环状序列处有 RNase R 富集、套索尾 RNase R 缺失以及分叉点处的非模板碱基。分叉点序列因其部分序列顺序与基因组注释相比稍显无序而与显后剪接序列类似。迄今为止,所有环状测序鉴定出的含有一真后剪接并被注释的丰富物种都是外显子环状

RNA。尽管环状测序可以产生深度环状及套索产物覆盖,但它亦有其局限性。这种方法比无需富集的测序法需要更多总 RNA 分子,并对内源性核酸酶污染更敏感。而且,它也或许与更长的环状 RNA 产物有偏倚。最终,核酸外切酶保护或许延伸至一些具有保护性 3′末端结构的线性产物中。

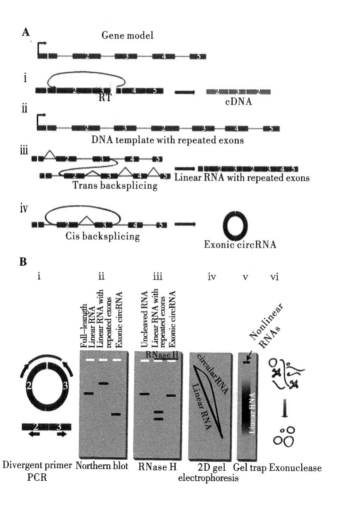

C

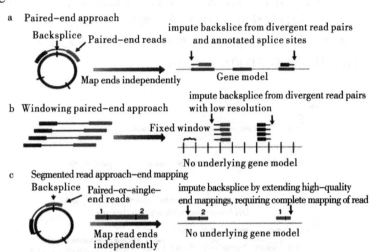

a Paired-end approach

Backsplice Paired-end reads

impute backslice from divergent read pairs
and annotated splice sites

Map ends independently Gene model

b Windowing paired-end approach

impute backsplice from divergent read pairs
with low resolution

Fixed window

No underlying gene model

c Segmented read approach-end mapping

Backsplice Paired-or-single-
end reads

impute backsplice by extending high-quality
end mappings, requiring complete mapping of read

Map read ends
independently

No underlying gene model

D

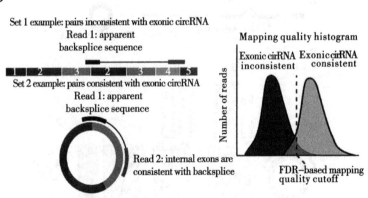

Set 1 example: pairs inconsistent with exonic circRNA

Read 1: apparent
backsplice sequence

Set 2 example: pairs consistent with exonic circRNA

Read 1: apparent
backsplice sequence

Read 2: internal exons are
consistent with backsplice

Mapping quality histogram

Exonic cirRNA
inconsistent

Exonic cirRNA
consistent

Number of reads

FDR-based mapping
quality cutoff

E

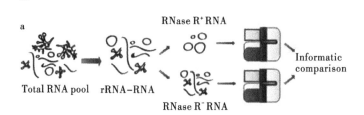

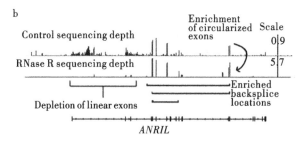

图 6 - 5 环状 RNA 分子的检测方法及其机制

（引自 Nat Biotechnol,2014,32:453 – 461）

三、环状 RNA 分子特征

环状 RNA 分子可由外显子（外显子 circRNAs）或者内含子（内含子 circRNAs）而来,因来源不同,形成机制不同,从而各具特征。Ivanov 等人发现环状 RNA 分子的产生具有一定规律可循,即根据两侧内含子是否含有逆向互补配对的基因组序列即可推断出环状 RNA 分子生成的基因位点（图 6 -6）。Reut Ashwal – Fluss 等人通过检测神经组织亦发现环状 RNA 分子为共同转录生成,生成速率主要由内含子序列决定。

Reverse complementary matches(RCMs) are a conserved feature of circRNA biogenesis

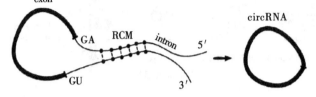

Computational analysis of intron sequences allows cirRNA prediction

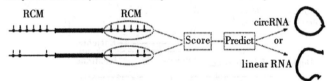

ADAR proteins antagonize circRNA biogenesis by "melting" the stem structure

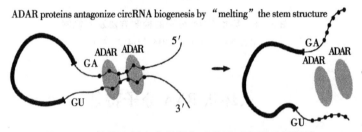

图 6 - 6　基因两侧内含子逆向互补配对序列对于环状

RNA 分子生成位点的推测意义

（引自 Cell Rep,2015,10:170 - 177）

（一）环状 RNA 分子结构特征概述

Laurent F. 等通过从 1000 个基因组计划进行单核苷酸多态性分析（SNP）发现：与相应的侧翼序列及随机位点相比，与 miRNA 结合的环状 RNA 分子种子位点的多态性显著下降，这一现象与和 miRNA 结合的 mRNA 分子 3′UTR 区种子位点多态性显著下降特征相一致,提示许多预测的环状 RNA 分子上与 miRNA 分子相结合的位点是具有功能的,并且如同 mRNA 与 miRNA 结合的位点一样,经历相似的选择压力。

外显子环状 RNA 在细胞中非常稳定,其大多数半衰期都在48 小时以上,而 mRNA 的平均半衰期仅仅 10 小时。然而,可能是循环 RNA 核酸外切酶的原因,外显子环状 RNA 在血浆中并不稳定,其半衰期不足 15 秒。细胞内的稳定性主要可能有赖于环状 RNA 对 RNA 核酸外切酶的抵抗作用。也许正是因为这种稳定性,通过测序读取计数方法及 qPCR 为基础的方法所得到的一些外显子环状 RNA 比线性 RNA 产物水平更高。外显子环状 RNA 并不包含 RNA 套索特征性的 2′—5′链接,因此可以抵抗 RNA 去分支酶的水解作用。若干不同的研究方法均显示:外显子环状 RNA 定位于细胞质,尽管目前对于细胞核输出过程还不甚清楚,估计环状 RNA 是在有丝分裂时从细胞核逸出至细胞质。外显子环状 RNA 对短干扰 RNA 介导的衰减亦非常敏感,这一特质对于研究其潜在功能具有较高价值。

外显子还有几个共有的序列为基础的特征。①迄今为止所发现的外显子环状 RNA 都涉及一 GT‐AG 经典剪接点碱基对。②外显子环状 RNA 几乎总是利用至少一个之前注释过的剪接点。涉及一后剪接的内含子侧翼位点倾向于比内含子长,但也有一些侧翼内含子比平均长度短些。内含子侧翼后剪接位点的互补序列似乎可以促进环化形成。尤其是,在倒置的后剪接点上下游的配对 Alu 重复序列在人外显子环状 RNA 形成位点处富集程度达五倍之多。同样,环状 RNA 过表达结构,包括互补上下游序列,相对于没有互补序列的结构而言,也显示了环状 RNA 形成的增强化。③外显子的长度可能会影响环化的形成,尤其是对仅由一个外显子构成的环状 RNA 来说。总体来说,基因组中促使环化形成的常常是超过平均长度的外显子,该外显子两侧是超过平均长度、含有易于促进内含子配对的串联重复序列内含子。

(二) 环状 RNA 的相对一致性

近年来,不同环状 RNA 全基因组研究发现彼此之间存在很大程度一致性。这些研究发现,在不同人类细胞类型中,存在上万种环状 RNA。将 rRNA 去除后进行测序数据统计,许多证实手段都表明 RNA 测序数据中的绝大部分显后剪接序列都来源于环状 RNA。相似的是,用类似方法分析小鼠 RNA 也发现了上万种环状转录本。大部分人类及小鼠环状 RNA 都来源于编码基因。对秀丽隐杆线虫的研究表明其有丰富的环状 RNA 且某些环状 RNA 具有生命周期调节功能。ENCODE 计划对人类细胞系进行的研究亦表明外显子环状 RNA 的生成受潜在线性 RNA 基因调节,且不同细胞间转录水平也不相同。哺乳动物外显子环状 RNA 的表达受调节控制以及具有高度保守性的特性说明这些转录本应该具有一定的功能。

由于很难单独从物理学角度上将环状 RNA 与线状 RNA 区分开,因此,环状 RNA 在总 RNA 池中的绝对丰度还很难度量。在环状 RNA 测序中应用的对照复制品中,一些后剪接产物的含量在 $1/300\,000\,000 \sim 1/300\,000$ 个读取。因此,若要分析环状 RNA,即使已经实施 RNase R 消化,至少需百万个读取,最好是亿万个。人们将配对末端读取与 qPCR 为基础的定量方法相结合,估算出外显子大约占多聚腺苷酸尾 RNA 总量的 1%,并且证实,外显子环状 RNA 包含了大量的非核糖体 RNA。

四、环状 RNA 的功能与潜在临床应用

环状 RNA 分子在人类细胞中含量丰富,且具有较高的保守

度,提示其或具有许多尚待发现的分子功能。譬如 William R. Jeck 等人在人成纤维细胞中发现了 25 000 种以上不同类型的环状 RNA 分子,并且这些分子与线性的 mRNA 相比具有更高的体内稳定性。

环状 RNA 在细胞中的丰度及进化保守性提示其可能在细胞生理学中具有一定功能,如结合 miRNA、结合蛋白、对翻译及翻译为蛋白质过程的调节等。

(一)潜在功能

1. miRNA 海绵

外显子环状 RNA 可与 miRNA 结合而充当"miRNA 海绵"的作用(图 6 - 7A,环状 RNA 作为 miRNA"海绵"示意图)。通过与相应 miRNA 结合,进而抑制 miRNA 与靶基因结合,从而提高相应编码 RNA 表达。譬如,外显子环状 RNA CDR1as 包含 74 个 miR - 7种子序列匹配,被 Argonaute 蛋白(该蛋白结合于 miRNA)紧密包围,miR - 7 以及 CDR1as 都在小鼠大脑中表达,体外显微镜下观察结果及免疫共沉淀实验表明二者具有相同的定位。敲除 CDR1as 或过表达曾被证实可裂解其的 miRNA,miR - 671 后,使得 miR - 7 靶基因的表达水平也相应下调;反之,CDR1as 过表达则可抑制 miR - 7 靶基因表达水平下调;而且,Qiupeng 等人亦发现,环状 RNA - HIPK3 可通过 18 个潜在结合位点与 9 个miRNA结合(图 6 - 8)。

2. 与 RNA 结合蛋白相互作用

之前的研究表明,某些线性非编码 RNA 转录本可隔绝 RNA 结合蛋白,外显子环状RNA 也有类似功能。譬如,环状 RNA 可稳定的与 AGO 蛋白及 RNA 聚合酶 Ⅱ 结合。外显子环状 RNA 也有某些作为 RNA 结合蛋白"支架"的特征,可与多种蛋白结合并通

过环状 RNA 转录本稳定性的增加而促进二者之间的结合。环状
RNA 亦可同时既和 RNA 结合蛋白结合,又和具有互补序列的
RNA 或 DNA 片段结合。并且,通过形成三级结构,环状 RNA 可
形成新的蛋白结合位点(图 6 - 7B,环状 RNA 作为 RNA 结合蛋白
调节因子发挥作用)。

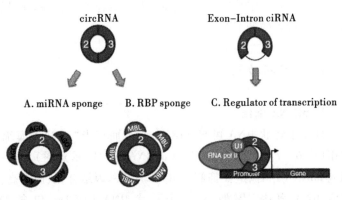

图 6 - 7　外显子环装 RNA 与 miRNA 结合的"海绵样"作用

(引自 Biochim Biophys Acta,2015,1859:163 - 168)

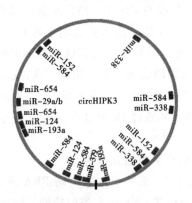

图 6 - 8　CircHIPK3 通过 18 个潜在结合位点与 9 个 miRNA 分子结合

(引自 Nat Commun,2016,7:11215)

3. 调节转录

环化机制可调节转录,譬如小鼠的 formin(Fmn)基因是肢体发育的关键基因,外显子环状 RNA 系通过一位于 Fmn 编码序列上游的剪接受体后剪接机制由 Fmn 转录本而产生。缺乏剪接受体的基因敲除小鼠因则不能检测出外显子环状 RNA 的表达,虽然其肢体发育正常,但是却有不完全渗透肾发育不全表型。不能从 Fmn 位点产生外显子环状 RNA 似乎导致 formin 蛋白的异常表达。即外显子环状 RNA 的形成通过隔绝转录起始位点发挥了类似于"mRNA 陷阱"的作用,进而产生一段非编码线性转录本并因此降低了 formin 蛋白表达水平(图 6 - 7C,环状 RNA 作调节转录作用机制示意图)。

4. 环状 RNA 的翻译

含有内核糖体契入位点(IRES)的环状 RNA 存在被翻译的可能性,尤其是具有 IRES 及 ATG 的环状 RNA。譬如一种乙型肝炎病毒的环状 RNA 卫星病毒环状 RNA hepatitis δ agent,可翻译出一种与致病性有关的病毒蛋白,但这种翻译机制并非经典机制,可能是某些病毒成分所特有。

5. 促使宿主基因转录

由内含子形成的"稳定环状内含子 RNA(ciRNA)"可与具有延伸功能的 RNA 聚合酶 II 结合从而促使宿主基因的转录(图 6 - 9)。

(二)潜在临床应用

Peifei Li 等应用 qRT - PCR 方法检测了 hsa_circ_002059 分子在 101 例胃癌及其癌旁组织中的表达,发现该分子在胃癌组织中的相对表达水平显著下调,与远处转移、TNM 分期、年龄等有关,并且术前、术后血浆中该分子表达水平也有显著差异,提出该分子或可作为胃癌潜在诊断标志物。

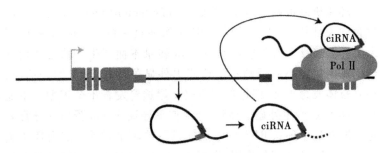

图6-9 ciRNA与RNA聚合酶Ⅱ结合促使宿主基因转录
（引自 Mol Cell,2013,51:705-706）

综上所述,外显子环状RNA具有潜在治疗靶点价值,假如采取合适的包装及输送方式的话,因其在细胞质中的高度稳定性,可长久对细胞生物学特性发挥调节功能。构建环状RNA过表达拟似物转染细胞可降低致癌miRNA分子的活性及功能。含有IRES序列的环状RNA可生成一些不常见的肽段,如长重复多聚肽等可用于合成新型生物材料。随着环状RNA更多新功能的发现,其用途也将日益广泛。

（王　颖）

参考文献

［1］ Ivanov A,Memczak S,Wyler E, et al. Analysis of intron sequences reveals hallmarks of circular RNA biogenesis in animals. Cell Rep, 2015, 10: 170-177.

［2］ Ashwal-Fluss R, Meyer M, Pamudurti NR, et al. circRNA biogenesis competes with pre-mRNA splicing. Mol Cell, 2014, 56: 55-66.

［3］ Zhang Y, Zhang XO, Chen T, et al. Circular intronic long noncoding

RNAs. Mol Cell, 2013, 51: 792 - 806.

[4] Memczak S, Jens M, Elefsinioti A, et al. Circular RNAs are a large class of animal RNAs with regulatory potency. Nature, 2013, 495: 333 - 338.

[5] Jeck WR, Sorrentino JA, Wang K, et al. Circular RNAs are abundant, conserved, and associated with ALU repeats. RNA, 2013, 19: 141 - 157.

[6] Salzman J, Gawad C, Wang PL, et al. Circular RNAs are the predominant transcript isoform from hundreds of human genes in diverse cell types. PLoS One, 2012, 7: e30733.

[7] Zhang XO, Wang HB, Zhang Y, et al. Complementary sequence - mediated exon circularization. Cell, 2014, 159: 134 - 147.

[8] Bentley DL. Coupling mRNA processing with transcription in time and space. Nat Rev Genet, 2014, 15: 163 - 175.

[9] Wilhelm BT, Marguerat S, Watt S, et al. Dynamic repertoire of a eukaryotic transcriptome surveyed at single - nucleotide resolution. Nature, 2008, 453: 1239 - 1243.

[10] Ebert MS, Sharp PA. Emerging roles for natural microRNA sponges. Curr Biol, 2010, 20: R858 - 861.

[11] Salzman J. Circular RNA expression: Its potential regulation and function. Trends Genet, 2016, 32: 309 - 316.

[12] Starke S, Jost I, Rossbach O, et al. Exon circularization requires canonical splice signals. Cell Rep, 2015, 10: 103 - 111.

[13] Burd CE, Jeck WR, Liu Y, et al. Expression of linear and novel circular forms of an INK4/ARF - associated non - coding RNA correlates with atherosclerosis risk. PLoS Genet, 2010, 6: e1001233.

[14] Corvelo A, Hallegger M, Smith CW, et al. Genome - wide association between branch point properties and alternative splicing. PLoS Comput Biol, 2010, 6: e1001016.

[15] Yang L, Duff MO, Graveley BR, et al. Genomewide characterization of non - polyadenylated RNAs. Genome Biol, 2011, 12: R16.

[16] Morten TV, Thomas BH, Susanne TV, et al. Spatio - temporal regulation of circular RNA expression during porcine embryonic brain development.

Genome Biol, 2014, 16: 1 – 17.

[17] Shen T, Han M, Wei G, et al. An intriguing RNA species—perspectives of circularized RNA. Protein Cell, 2015, 6: 871 – 880.

[18] Hansen TB, Wiklund ED, Bramsen JB, et al. miRNA – dependent gene silencing involving Ago2 – mediated cleavage of a circular antisense RNA. EMBO J, 2011, 30: 4414 – 4422.

[19] Graveley BR. Molecular biology: power sequencing. Nature, 2008, 453: 1197 – 1198.

[20] Hansen TB, Jensen TI, Clausen BH, et al. Natural RNA circles function as efficient microRNA sponges. Nature, 2013, 495: 384 – 388.

[21] Chen I, Chen CY, Chuang TJ. Biogenesis, identification, and function of exonic circular RNAs. Wiley Interdiscip Rev RNA, 2015, 6:563 – 579.

[22] Hu GJ, Chen J, Zhao XN, et al. Production of ACAT1 56kDa isoform in human cells via trans – splicing involving the ampicillin resistance gene. Cell Res, 2013, 23:1007 – 1024.

[23] Cocquet J, Chong A, Zhang G, et al. Reverse transcriptase template switching and false alternative transcripts. Genomics, 2006, 88:127 – 131.

[24] Conn S, Pillman K, Toubia J, et al. The RNA binding protein quaking regulates formation of circRNAs. Cell, 2015, 160: 1125 – 1134.

[25] Iverfeldt K, Serfözö P, Diaz AL, et al. RNA circularization strategies in vivo and in vitro. Nucleic Acids Res, 2015, 43: 2454 – 2465.

[26] Wang Y, Wang Z. Efficientbacksplicing produces translatable circular mRNAs. RNA, 2015, 21: 172 – 179.

[27] Ashwal – Fluss R, Meyer M, Pamudurti NR, et al. circRNA biogenesis competes with pre – mRNA splicing. Mol Cell, 2014, 56: 55 – 66.

[28] Ahmed I, Karedath T, Andrews SS, et al. Altered expression pattern of circular RNAs in primary and metastatic sites of epithelial ovarian carcinoma. Oncotarget, 2016, 7: 36366 – 36381

[29] Li X, Zhao L, Jiang H, et al. Short homologous sequences are strongly associated with the generation of chimeric RNAs in eukaryotes. J Mol Evol, 2009, 68: 56 – 65.

[30] Dobin A, Davis CA, Schlesinger F, et al. STAR: ultrafast universal RNA – seq aligner. Bioinformatics, 2013, 29:15 – 21.

[31] Buratti E, Baralle FE. TDP – 43: new aspects of autoregulation mechanisms in RNA binding proteins and their connection with human disease. FEBS J, 2011, 278: 3530 – 3538.

[32] Danan M, Schwartz S,Edelheit S, et al. Transcriptome – wide discovery of circular RNAs in Archaea. Nucleic Acids Res, 2012, 40: 3131 – 3142.

[33] Lu D, Xu AD. Mini review: CircularRNAs as potential clinical biomarkers for disorders in the central nervous system. Front Genet, 2016, 7: 53.

[34] Engreitz JM, Pandya – Jones A, McDonel P, et al. The Xist lncRNA exploits three – dimensional genome architecture to spread across the X chromosome. Science, 2013, 341: 1237973.

[35] Ebbesen KK, Kjems J, Hansen TB. Circular RNAs: identification, biogenesis and function. Biochimica Et Biophysica Acta, 2015, 1859: 163 – 168.

[36] Zheng Q, Bao C, Guo W, et al. Circular RNA profiling reveals an abundantcircHIPK3 that regulates cell growth by sponging multiple miRNAs. Nat Commun, 2016, 7: 11215.

第七章

针对前列腺特异性膜抗原的人源性抗体偶联药物研究

前列腺癌(prostate cancer, PCa)是严重威胁男性健康的常见泌尿系肿瘤。在西方国家,前列腺癌占男性癌症死因的第二位。在我国随着生活水平的提高、饮食习惯的改变以及人口老龄化问题的凸显,前列腺癌的发病率也逐年升高。目前手术治疗、放疗、内分泌治疗等是主要的治疗策略,且都取得了一定的进展,但临床上在接受前列腺癌根治术的患者中仍有27%～53%在术后十年内会发生肿瘤的局部复发或远处转移,而以内分泌治疗为主的激素敏感性前列腺癌患者,最终几乎都会发展为激素非依赖性前列腺癌。这些是传统治疗方法所不能解决的问题。因此,迫切需要寻找新的治疗方法。

前列腺特异性膜抗原(prostate specific membrane antigen, PSMA)是一种表达于前列腺上皮细胞的Ⅱ型跨膜糖蛋白,PSMA含有多个抗原表位,可与多种单克隆抗体结合,是进行前列腺癌靶向治疗的有效靶点。由于PSMA在前列腺肿瘤细胞及其转移灶中的表达明显高于正常前列腺上皮细胞,此外,PSMA在多种实体肿瘤的新生血管内皮细胞上也有表达,但在正常的血管内皮细胞上却不表达,因此,PSMA是一种理想的肿瘤治疗靶点。

近一百年间,基于抗体的免疫疗法和基于化学药物的化学疗法一直是临床上肿瘤治疗的两大策略。在临床实践中,治疗性抗体虽然靶向性强,但由于其分子量大、穿透性差,因此对于实体瘤的治疗效果有限。小分子化学药物虽然具备对癌细胞的高度杀伤效力,但也常常误伤正常细胞,引起严重的副作用。抗体偶联药物(antibody – drug conjugate, ADC)由抗体、化学药物及"连接肽"(linker)共同构成,它能协同发挥抗体药物和化学药物的优点,实现对肿瘤细胞的特异性杀伤,是非常有前景的抗肿瘤药物。

一、抗体偶联药物的研究进展

由于抗体具有特异性强,靶向性好等特点,使得抗体偶联药物成为肿瘤治疗的重要方法。抗体偶联药物能有效避免传统化疗药物对肿瘤细胞的非特异性杀伤。目前,常用于 ADC 的药物有 18 种。这 18 种药物可以分为两大类:一类是微管抑制剂如 Auristatin(如 MMAE 及 MMAF)和 Maytansinoid(如 DM1 及 DM4),另一类是 DNA 断裂剂(如卡里奇霉素)。Maytansinoid 是美登素的衍生物,它和 Auristatin 是目前应用最多的是微管抑制剂类的两种代表药物。

(一)偶联美登素的抗体偶联药物研究进展

美登素是从非洲灌木树皮中分离得到的。美登素及其衍生物 DM1 和 DM4 能与细胞的微管结合,造成细胞有丝分裂阻滞,从而发挥其毒性作用。美登素与抗体偶联要选择合适的连接方法,用于连接美登素的 linker 有两种:不可切割 linker 和可切割 linker。目前最常用也最成熟的连接方式是采用不可切割、用硫醚键连接的方法,其与可切割 linker 相比具有更高的连接效率,此外,其可通过细胞的内体转运途径,更容易被水解,从而有效释放抗体所偶联的药物。

针对 HER2 的抗体偶联药物 Trastuzumab – DM1(T – DM1)是

在 Trastuzumab 基础上通过 SMCC 与微管抑制剂 DM1 偶联制备而成的,T-DM1 于 2013 年被 FDA 批准用于晚期 HER2 阳性转移性乳腺癌的治疗。Jumbe 等在乳腺癌动物模型中证实 T-DM1 能够明显抑制 HER2 阳性乳腺癌的生长。Lewis 等通过建立 HER2 阳性乳腺癌移植瘤模型,证实 T-DM1 能够显著抑制 HER2 阳性肿瘤的生长。Barok 等发现,在体外 T-DM1 能够特异性杀伤 HER2 阳性的胃癌细胞,在荷瘤裸鼠体内给予 T-DM1 治疗,也能明显抑制肿瘤生长。Junttila 等发现对 lapatinib 抵抗的 HER2 阳性乳腺癌荷瘤裸鼠给予 T-DM1 治疗后,肿瘤明显缩小,具有明显的抑瘤作用。Borges 等对 HER2 阳性乳腺癌伴脑转移患者给予放射治疗并同时给予 T-DM1 治疗,联合治疗 6 个月后,MRI 检测发现不论是肿瘤原发灶还是肿瘤转移部位均未检测出肿瘤。Yu 等用 HER2 阳性的卵巢癌细胞接种裸鼠建立移植瘤模型,在给予 T-DM1 治疗后发现,T-DM1 能够明显抑制肿瘤生长,具有良好的抑瘤效果。

AVE9633 是由抗 CD33 的人源化抗体 huMy9 与 DM4 偶联后制备而成的。在 I 期临床试验中,AVE9633 能够显著抑制慢性白血病细胞的生长,具有显著的治疗效果。

(二)偶联 Auristatin 的抗体偶联药物研究进展

Auristatin 是全化学合成的药物,相对容易改造,便于优化其物理性质和成药。目前,用于进行抗体偶联的主要是 Auristatin 的衍生物包括 Auristatin E(MMAE)和 Auristatin F(MMAF)。MMAE 可在低浓度下抑制多种肿瘤细胞的生长,但是毒性相对较大。为了降低 MMAE 的细胞毒性,在 MMAE 的结构基础上改造出了另一种优化的衍生物 MMAF,它降低了 MMAE 的毒性,但是这也导致 MMAF 穿过细胞膜的能力变差,使其对细胞的杀伤活性有所下降。

Li 等用抗 CD22 的人源化抗体通过 MC – vc – PAB linker 与 MMAE 偶联制备得到抗体偶联药物,将其命名为 DCDT2980S,在用非霍奇金淋巴瘤细胞建立的动物模型中,DCDT2980S 能显著抑制肿瘤细胞的生长。多发性骨髓细胞高表达 FcRL5,Elkins 等将抗 FcRL5 的抗体与 MMAE 进行偶联制备出抗体偶联药物 anti – FcRL5 – MC – vcPAB – MMAE,在荷瘤裸鼠模型中证实该药物能够显著抑制骨髓瘤细胞的生长。Gerber 等将抗 CD19 的 hBU12 抗体与 MMAE 偶联制备得到了抗体偶联药物 hBU12 – vcMMAE。hBU12 – vcMMAE 能够显著抑制 Rituximab 不敏感的淋巴瘤细胞生长。Li 等将抗 CD20 的抗体 Ofatumumab 与 MMAE 偶联制备出抗体偶联药物 OFA – vcMMAE,发现其能特异性内化入 CD20 阳性的白血病 K562 细胞中,在胞内溶酶体酶的作用下,MMAE 从抗体上释放,诱导肿瘤细胞凋亡,此外,在荷瘤裸鼠体内也具有明显的抑瘤效果。Dornan 等将抗 CD79d 的人源化抗体与 MMAE 偶联,发现制备出的抗体偶联药物能显著抑制淋巴瘤细胞的生长。组织因子(tissue factor,TF)在多种实体肿瘤细胞表面高表达,Breij 等设计出针对 TF 的抗体偶联药物 TF – 011 – MMAE,并用不同类型的肿瘤组织接种裸鼠建立了患者来源的移植瘤模型(patient – derived xenograft,PDX),给予 TF – 011 – MMAE 治疗后,发现能有效抑制患者来源的 TF 阳性胰腺癌、非小细胞肺癌和前列腺癌的生长。

Jackson 等将抗 EphA2 受体的人源性抗体 1C1 与微管抑制剂 MMAF 偶联制备出抗体偶联药物 1C1 – mcMMAF,每周给荷瘤裸鼠注射 1mg/kg 的抗体偶联药物,发现能显著抑制肿瘤的生长。Oflazoglu 等将抗 CD70 的人源化抗体 h1F6 与 MMAF 偶联后,发现该 ADC 在体内外均能显著抑制恶性胶质瘤和肾细胞癌的生长。

综上所述,由于抗体偶联药物能够特异性地将药物带到肿瘤细胞内从而发挥对肿瘤细胞的靶向性杀伤,使得抗体偶联药物越来越受到研究者的关注。目前,随着更多的肿瘤靶点被发现,相信会有更多的抗体偶联药物被研发用于肿瘤的靶向治疗。

二、以 PSMA 为靶点的前列腺癌靶向治疗的研究进展

2013 年,抗体介导的肿瘤免疫治疗被美国《科学》杂志评为十大科学进展之首。抗体介导的肿瘤免疫治疗的关键是要找到合适的靶点。在前列腺癌的免疫治疗中也不例外。前列腺特异性膜抗原(prostate specific membrane antigen,PSMA)是一种表达于前列腺上皮细胞的 II 型跨膜糖蛋白,是一种具有叶酸水解酶和神经羧肽酶活性的酶分子,分子量为 100 kDa。PSMA 由 750 个氨基酸组成,分为三个结构域,其氨基端位于细胞膜内,含有 19 个氨基酸(氨基酸序列 1 ~ 19),跨膜区含有 24 个氨基酸(氨基酸序列 20 ~ 44),膜外区含有 705 个氨基酸(氨基酸序列 45 ~ 750),其胞内区和胞外区含有多个抗原表位,可与多种单克隆抗体结合,使得这些抗体具有良好的应用前景。由于 PSMA 在前列腺肿瘤细胞及其转移灶中的表达明显高于正常前列腺上皮细胞,此外,PSMA 在多种实体肿瘤的新生血管内皮细胞上也有表达,但在正常血管内皮细胞上却不表达,使其成为一种理想的肿瘤治疗靶点。

(一)针对 PSMA 的抗体研究进展

由于单克隆抗体具有特异性高、稳定性好并可大量生产的特

点,使得抗 PSMA 的单克隆抗体也成为国内外研究的热点。PSMA为跨膜糖蛋白,根据抗体与 PSMA 结合部位的不同,可将抗体分为两大类:一类是针对 PSMA 胞内区的抗体,另一类是针对 PSMA 胞外区的抗体。

在胞内区抗体中,目前以 7E11. C5 单抗的研究最多,该抗体也是应用最早的 PSMA 单抗。该抗体与胞内区 N - 末端的线性表位结合,因此不能与活细胞结合。PM2J004. 5 是另一种针对 PSMA胞内区的抗体,其识别表位也是线性表位,IHC 检测发现, PM2J004. 5 与 PSMA 的结合能力较 7E11. C5 强。

目前研究更多的还是针对 PSMA 胞外区的抗体。例如 J591、J533、E99 等。Murphy 等的研究发现,3F5. 4G6 与 PSMA 胞外区的不同表位结合,它们可与 LNCaP 活细胞特异性结合,而不与变性的 PSMA 结合,因此不能用于 Western blot 检测,这些抗体所识别的表位为构象表位。由于这些抗体可与活细胞结合,因此,这些针对 PSMA 胞外区的抗体更适合用于靶向治疗的研究。

(二)针对 PSMA 的 ADC 研究进展

目前,以 PSMA 为治疗靶点的抗体偶联药物陆续被报道,均显示出了明显的治疗效果。Wang 等在抗 PSMA 的抗体上偶联 Auristatin,构建成针对 PSMA 的 ADC,用于前列腺癌的治疗,证实其能有效杀伤 PSMA 阳性前列腺癌细胞,而对 PSMA 阴性细胞则无明显影响。Ma 等也利用针对 PSMA 的抗体偶联药物 PSMA - MMAE 治疗 C4 - 2 荷瘤裸鼠,发现用 ADC 治疗后的裸鼠,生存时间是未治疗组的 9 倍,且有 40% 的荷瘤裸鼠体内的肿瘤完全消失。Murga 等证实 PSMA - MMAE 能够有效抑制雄激素依赖性和非依赖性前列腺癌的生长,并延长裸鼠的生存时间。DiPippo 等将抗 PSMA 的抗体与 MMAE 进行偶联,成功制备出了另一种

PSMA – ADC,并证实其在体内可特异性抑制 PSMA 阳性肿瘤的生长,并延长荷瘤裸鼠的生存时间,此外他们还发现 PSMA – MMAE 治疗的裸鼠血清中 PSA 的水平明显降低,提示 PSMA – MMAE 对前列腺癌具有明显的抑制作用。此外,该学者用患者的前列腺癌组织接种裸鼠建立了 PDX 模型,并给予 PSMA – MMAE 进行治疗,发现能有效抑制患者来源的 PSMA 阳性前列腺癌的生长,并明显延长裸鼠的生存时间。

随着研究的不断深入,MLN2704(即针对 PSMA 胞外区的抗体 J591 偶联 DM1)已经完成Ⅰ期临床试验。结果显示,其可成功抑制肿瘤的生长,并且副作用低,证实了其安全性。

综上所述,PSMA 是一个理想的抗肿瘤治疗靶点,以 PSMA 为治疗靶点的抗体偶联药物具有良好的应用前景。

本课题组从酵母展示 scFv 抗体库中筛选获得一株抗 PSMA 的单链抗体,我们将其的轻、重链可变区基因分别与恒定区序列拼接,获得完整的抗体轻、重链基因,并对基因序列进行了密码子优化,使其能够在 CHO 细胞中高表达,将优化后的抗体轻、重链基因进行合成后分别克隆入真核表达载体 pCDNA3,获得抗体轻、重链的表达载体,分别命名为 pCDNA3 – LC 和 pCDNA3 – HC。将轻、重链表达质粒按照 4:1 的比例瞬时转染 CHO – S 细胞进行表达,收集培养上清液,利用亲和层析柱进行纯化,获得抗 PSMA 的全抗体,将其命名为 PSMAb。我们利用细胞 ELISA、间接免疫荧光染色和流式细胞术检测了 PSMAb 的亲和力、内化活性及其与 PSMA 阳性细胞的结合能力。我们将 PSMAb 与近红外染料 IRDye 800CW 偶联后,注射给 PSMA 阳性和 PSMA 阴性的荷瘤裸鼠,检测其在体内的分布情况。我们将 PSMAb 与微管抑制剂 DM1 进行偶联,制备出抗体偶联药物 PSMAb – DM1,并在体内外验证了其对 PSMA 阳性肿瘤细胞的特异性杀伤活性。

我们的结果显示,PSMAb 抗体轻、重链的真核表达载体构建成功。将它们瞬时转染 CHO - S 细胞后可有效表达 PSMAb,亲和层析获得了纯度较高的 PSMAb 蛋白。细胞 ELISA、流式细胞术及间接免疫荧光染色等实验证实 PSMAb 具有高亲和力,能特异性地与 PSMA 阳性细胞结合,并可有效内化入 PSMA 阳性细胞。体内实验发现,IRDye 800CW 标记的 PSMAb 可特异性分布于 PSMA 阳性肿瘤组织。

之后,我们将 PSMAb 与 DM1 偶联,流式细胞术证实 DM1 的偶联不影响 PSMAb 与 PSMA 阳性细胞的结合能力,间接免疫荧光染色证实 PSMAb - DM1 仍可有效内化入 PSMA 阳性细胞。在体外利用 Alamar Blue 实验和凋亡检测,我们证实 PSMAb - DM1 可有效杀伤 PSMA 阳性细胞,并可诱导 PSMA 阳性细胞凋亡。计算得出 PSMAb - DM1 的 IC50 浓度为 0.12 nmol/L。体内实验证实 PSMAb - DM1 可有效抑制 PSMA 阳性肿瘤的生长。

综上所述,我们的研究:①成功构建了抗 PSMA 人源性抗体 PSMAb 轻、重链的真核表达载体;②瞬时转染 CHO - S 细胞后,利用亲和层析的方法获得了高纯度的 PSMAb 抗体;③细胞 ELISA、流式细胞术和间接免疫荧光染色证实 PSMAb 具有高亲和力,可特异性结合并有效内化入 PSMA 阳性肿瘤细胞;④将 PSMAb 与 DM1 偶联后,成功制备出抗体偶联药物 PSMAb - DM1;⑤证实 PSMAb - DM1 可在体外特异性杀伤 PSMA 阳性肿瘤细胞,可在体内有效抑制 PSMA 阳性肿瘤的生长。这些研究为该抗体的进一步应用奠定了基础。

(吴介恒　温伟红)

参考文献

[1]　Siegel RL, Miller KD,Jemal A. Cancer statistics, 2015. CA Cancer J Clin,

2015, 65: 5 – 29.

[2] Chang SS. Overview of prostate – specific membrane antigen. Rev Urol, 2004, 6: S13 – 18.

[3] Remillard S, Rebhun LI, Howie GA, et al. Antimitotic activity of the potent tumor inhibitor maytansine. Science, 1975, 189: 1002 – 1005.

[4] Mandelbaum – Shavit F, Wolpert – DeFilippes MK, Johns DG. Binding of maytansine to rat brain tubulin. Biochem Biophys Res Commun, 1976, 72: 47 – 54.

[5] Bhattacharyya B, Wolff J. Maytansine binding to the vinblastine sites of tubulin. FEBS Lett, 1977, 75: 159 – 162.

[6] Austin CD, Wen X, Gazzard L, et al. Oxidizing potential of endosomes and lysosomes limits intracellular cleavage of disulfide – based antibody – drug conjugates. Proc Natl Acad Sci USA, 2005, 102(50): 17987 – 17992.

[7] Lewis Phillips GD, Li G, Dugger DL, et al. Targeting HER2 – positive breast cancer with trastuzumab – DM1, an antibody – cytotoxic drug conjugate. Cancer Res, 2008, 68: 9280 – 9290.

[8] Krop I, Winer EP. Trastuzumab emtansine: a novel antibody – drug conjugate for HER2 – positive breast cancer. Clin Cancer Res, 2014, 20: 15 – 20.

[9] Jumbe NL, Xin Y, Leipold DD, et al. Modeling the efficacy of trastuzu mab – DM1, an antibody drug conjugate, in mice. J Pharmacokinet Pharmacodyn, 2010, 37: 221 – 242.

[10] Barok M, Tanner M, Koninki K, et al. Trastuzumab – DM1 is highly effective in preclinical models of HER2 – positive gastric cancer. Cancer Lett, 2011, 306: 171 – 179.

[11] Junttila TT, Li G, Parsons K, et al. Trastuzumab – DM1 (T – DM1) ret ains all the mechanisms of action of trastuzumab and efficiently inhibits growth of lapatinib insensitive breast cancer. Breast Cancer Res Treat, 2011, 128: 347 – 356.

[12] Borges GS, Rovere RK, Dias SM, et al. Safety and efficacy of the combination of T – DM1 with radiotherapy of the central nervous system in a patient with HER2 – positive metastatic breast cancer: case study and re-

view of the literature. Ecancermedicalscience, 2015, 9: 586.

[13] Yu L, Wang Y, Yao Y, et al. Eradication of growth of HER2 - positive ovarian cancer withtrastuzumab - DM1, an antibody - cytotoxic drug conjugate in mouse xenograft model. Int J Gynecol Cancer, 2014, 24:1158 - 1164.

[14] Laszlo GS, Estey EH, Walter RB. The past and future of CD33 as therapeutic target in acute myeloid leukemia. Blood Rev, 2014, 28: 143 - 153.

[15] Lapusan S, Vidriales MB, Thomas X, et al. Phase I studies of AVE9633, an anti - CD33 antibody - maytansinoid conjugate, in adult patients with relapsed/refractory acute myeloid leukemia. Invest New Drugs, 2012, 30: 1121 - 1131.

[16] Carter PJ, Senter PD. Antibody - drug conjugates for cancer therapy. Cancer J, 2008, 14: 154 - 169.

[17] Doronina SO, Mendelsohn BA, Bovee TD, et al. Enhanced activity of monomethylauristatin F through monoclonal antibody delivery: effects of linker technology on efficacy and toxicity. Bioconjug Chem, 2006, 17: 114 - 124.

[18] Li D, Poon KA, Yu SF, et al. DCDT2980S, an anti - CD22 - monomethylauristatin E antibody - drug conjugate, is a potential treatment for non - Hodgkin lymphoma. Mol Cancer Ther, 2013, 12: 1255 - 1265.

[19] Elkins K, Zheng B, Go M, et al. FcRL5 as a target of antibody - drug conjugates for the treatment of multiple myeloma. Mol Cancer Ther, 2012, 11: 2222 - 2232.

[20] Gerber HP, Kung - Sutherland M, Stone I, et al. Potent antitumor activity of the anti - CD19 auristatin antibody drug conjugate hBU12 - vcM-MAE against rituximab - sensitive and - resistant lymphomas. Blood, 2009, 113: 4352 - 4361.

[21] Li ZH, Zhang Q, Wang HB, et al. Preclinical studies of targeted therapies for CD20 - positive B lymphoid malignancies byOfatumumab conjugated with auristatin. Invest New Drugs, 2014, 32: 75 - 86.

[22] Dornan D, Bennett F, Chen Y, et al. Therapeutic potential of an anti - CD79b antibody - drug conjugate, anti - CD79b - vc - MMAE, for the

treatment of non – Hodgkin lymphoma. Blood, 2009, 114: 2721 – 2729.

[23] Breij EC, de Goeij BE, Verploegen S, et al. An antibody – drug conjugate that targets tissue factor exhibits potent therapeutic activity against a broad range of solid tumors. Cancer Res, 2014, 74: 1214 – 1226.

[24] Jackson D, Gooya J, Mao S, et al. A human antibody – drug conjugate targeting EphA2 inhibits tumor growth in vivo. Cancer Res, 2008, 68: 9367 – 9374.

[25] Oflazoglu E, Stone IJ, Gordon K, et al. Potent anticarcinoma activity of the humanized anti – CD70 antibody h1F6 conjugated to the tubulin inhibitor auristatin via an uncleavable linker. Clin Cancer Res, 2008, 14: 6171 – 6180.

[26] Israeli RS, Powell CT, Fair WR, et al. Molecular cloning of a complementary DNA encoding a prostate – specific membrane antigen. Cancer Res, 1993, 53: 227 – 230.

[27] Marchal C, Redondo M, Padilla M, et al. Expression of prostate specific membrane antigen (PSMA) in prostatic adenocarcinoma and prostatic intraepithelial neoplasia. Histol Histopathol, 2004, 19: 715 – 718.

[28] Liu H, Moy P, Kim S, et al. Monoclonal antibodies to the extracellular domain of prostate – specific membrane antigen also react with tumor vascular endothelium. Cancer Res, 1997, 57: 3629 – 3634.

[29] Baccala A, Sercia L, Li J, et al. Expression of prostate – specific membrane antigen in tumor – associated neovasculature of renal neoplasms. Urology, 2007, 70: 385 – 390.

[30] Chang SS, Reuter VE, Heston WD, et al. Five different anti – prostate – specific membrane antigen (PSMA) antibodies confirm PSMA expression in yumor – associated neovasculature. Cancer Res, 1999, 59: 3192 – 3198.

[31] Sweat SD, Pacelli A, Murphy GP, et al. Prostate – specific membrane antigen expression is greatest in prostate adenocarcinoma and lymph node metastases. Urology, 1998, 52: 637 – 640.

[32] Wright GL Jr, Grob BM, Haley C, et al. Upregulation of prostate – specific membrane antigen after androgen – deprivation therapy. Urology, 1996,

48: 326 - 334.

[33] Chang SS, Reuter VE, Heston WD, et al. Metastatic renal cell carcinoma neovasculature expresses prostate - specific membrane antigen. Urology, 2001, 57: 801 - 805.

[34] Murphy GP, Greene TG, Tino WT, et al. Isolation and characterization of monoclonal antibodies specific for the extracellular domain of prostate specific membrane antigen. J Urol, 1998, 160: 2396 - 2401.

[35] Tino WT, Huber MJ, Lake TP, et al. Isolation and characterization of monoclonal antibodies specific for protein conformational epitopes present in prostate - specific membrane antigen (PSMA). Hybridoma, 2000, 19: 249 - 257.

[36] Murphy GP, Kenny GM, Ragde H, et al. Measurement of serum prostate - specific membrane antigen, a new prognostic marker for prostate cancer. Urology, 1998, 51: 89 - 97.

[37] Wang X, Ma D, Olson WC, et al. In vitro and in vivo responses of advanced prostate tumors to PSMA ADC, an auristatin - conjugated antibody to prostate - specific membrane antigen. Mol Cancer Ther, 2011, 10: 1728 - 1739.

[38] Ma D, Hopf CE, Malewicz AD, et al. Potent antitumor activity of an auristatin - conjugated, fully human monoclonal antibody to prostate - specific membrane antigen. Clin Cancer Res, 2006, 12: 2591 - 2596.

[39] Murga JD, Moorji SM, Han AQ, et al. Synergistic co - targeting of prostate - specific membrane antigen and androgen receptor in prostate cancer. Prostate, 2015, 75: 242 - 254.

[40] DiPippo VA, Olson WC, Nguyen HM, et al. Efficacy studies of an antibody - drug conjugate PSMA - ADC in patient - derived prostate cancer xenografts. Prostate, 2015, 75: 303 - 313.

[41] DiPippo VA, Nguyen HM, Brown LG, et al. Addition of PSMA ADC to enzalutamide therapy significantly improves survival in in vivo model of castration resistant prostate cancer. Prostate, 2015, 76: 325 - 334.

[42] Henry MD, Wen S, Silva MD, et al. A prostate - specific membrane anti-

gen – targeted monoclonal antibody – chemotherapeutic conjugate designed for the treatment of prostate cancer. Cancer Res, 2004, 64: 7995 – 8001.

[43] Galsky MD, Eisenberger M, Moore – Cooper S, et al. Phase I trial of the prostate – specific membrane antigen – directed immunoconjugate MLN2704 in patients with progressive metastatic castration – resistant prostate cancer. J Clin Oncol, 2008, 26: 2147 – 2154.

[44] Brand TC, Tolcher AW. Management of high risk metastatic prostate cancer: the case for novel therapies. J Urol, 2006, 176: S76 – 80.

综述一

Targeted therapy in esophageal cancer

Abstract

An increasing number of patients are diagnosed with esophageal cancer at advanced stages, and only a small group of them can benefit from the traditional chemotherapy and radiotherapy. So far, multiple monoclonal antibodies and tyrosine kinase inhibitors have been developed, alone or in combination with traditional therapy, to improve the prognosis of patients with advanced esophageal cancer. This review summarizes the recent advances of targeted therapies against EGFR, HER2, VEGFR and c – MET in esophageal cancer. More clinical trials should be performed to evaluate the efficacy and safety of various targeted therapy regimens. Future basic research should focus on investigating the molecular mechanisms of therapeutic targets in esophageal cancer.

Key words: Esophageal cancer; Targeted therapy; EGFR; HER2; VEGFR; c – MET

1. Introduction

Esophageal cancer is the eighth most common cancer and the sixth leading cause of cancer – related mortality in the world. Esophageal cancer consists of two main histological types: squamous cell cancer, which is the predominant type, and adenocarcinoma, whose incidence is rapidly increasing in western European countries. The poor nutritional status, low intake of fruits and vegetables, and drinking beverages at high temperatures are regarded as main risk factors for esophageal squamous cell cancer, while the primary risk factors of esophageal adenocarcinoma are overweight, obesity and chronic gastroesophageal reflux disease.

For localized esophageal cancer, surgery remains the primary treatment. However, even after radical resection the majority of patients recur in regional or distant sites with a 5 - year survival rate of only 20% ~ 25%. Primary radiotherapy shows the advantage of avoidance of perioperative morbidity and mortality, but also brings about catastrophic local and regional complications such as esophagotracheal fistulas. For patients with locally advanced and metastatic disease, the main treatment is a combination of two or three chemotherapy agents, such as irinotecan, fluorouracil and taxane. It is reported that the addition of a third agent into a two - drug regimen has slightly improved the survival rate, but with a remarkable additional toxicity, which is hardly acceptable to the elderly patients. Therefore, there is a critical need to develop new effective agents able to give a survival benefit with acceptable tolerability.

Recently, with increasing insights into the molecular mechanism of esophageal cancer, a variety of molecular targeted agents have been developed. Here we review the advances of epidermal growth factor receptor (EGFR), human epidermal growth factor receptor (HER2), vascular endothelial growth factor (VEGR) and mesenchymal - epithelial transition factor receptor targeted therapies in esophageal cancer, and analyze the problems existing in these therapies.

2. EGFR targeted therapy

EGFR family consists of four members: ErbB1, ErbB2, ErbB3 and ErbB4. EGFR is a 170kDa glycoprotein, and involves a large extracellular region, a single spanning transmembrane domain, an intracellular juxtamembrane region, a tyrosine kinase domain and a C - terminal regulatory region. Multiple ligands, including epidermal growth factor, transforming growth factor - alpha, amphiregulin, heparin binding - EGF, epiregulin and betacellulin can activate EGFR by binding to its extracellular domain, resulting in the phosphorylation of the intracellular tyrosine kinases. Activation of EGFR may trigger a series of intracellular signaling pathways, such as Ras/Raf/MAPK and AKT/mTOR pathways, which play important roles in cell proliferation, apoptosis, angiogenesis and metastasis.

EGFR is constitutively expressed on the surface of various cell types, such as epithelial cells, gliocytes, fibroblasts and keratinocytes. EGFR overexpression occurs in 60% ~70% even to 95.2% esophageal squamous cell cancer patients, and is associated with higher depth of invasion, vascular invasion, and poor prognosis. EGFR targeted therapies consist of two main classes: monoclonal antibodies (mAbs) and tyrosine kinase inhibitors (TKIs).

2.1 Anti - EGFRmAbs

EGFR mAbs, firstly developed in advanced colorectal cancer, mainly involve four types: cetuximab, panitumumab, nimotuzumab and matuzumab.

Cetuximab, originally derived from a mouse myeloma cell line, is an IgG1 mAb that blocks EGFR activation. It is one of the first two anti - EGFR mAbs approved for the treatment of metastatic colorectal cancer, either as single agent or in combination with chemotherapy. It is also effective in other cancers, such as the head and neck cancer and non – small cell lung cancer.

In esophageal cancer, the efficacy and safety of cetuximab have been evaluated in many clinical trials. Firstly, it has been widely studied in combination with chemotherapy. It was reported that cetuximab combined with pemetrexed was marginally effective and well tolerated in advanced esophageal squamous cell cancer patients as the second – line treatmen. Oxaliplatin, fluorouracil and leucovorin (FOLFOX) plus cetuximab was proved as a safe and effective neoadjuvant therapy for synchronous advanced rectal and esophageal cancer. For treating patients with docetaxel – refractory esophagogastric cancer, the combination of cetuximab and docetaxel achieved modest response rate with low incidence of toxicity. However, sometimes insufferable toxicities also occurred. In a prospective clinical trial, adding preoperative cetuximab and radiotherapy to perioperative epirubicin, cisplatin, and capecitabine (ECX) chemotherapy was well tolerated and did not interfere with the resectability rate (100%) in patients with esophageal adenocarcinoma, but the high incidence (50%) of postoperative serious adverse events probably caused by perioperative ECX ended this study prematurely. Secondly, cetuximab has been evaluated in combination with radiotherapy. In a open – label, single – arm, multicenter study of patients with surgically resectable esophageal and gastrioesophageal junction carcinomas, cetuximab combined with radiation therapy showed a comparable pathologic complete response (pCR) rate and a better toxicity rate compared with preoperative chemotherapy and radiation therapy. In another clinical study, cetuximab plus docetaxel and oxaliplatin improved the response

rate minimally, but failed to improve the progression – free survival
(PFS), overall survival (OS) and 1 – year survival. Thirdly, cetuximab has been tested in esophageal cancer in combination with chemoradiotherapy. In a prospective, multicenter trial, cetuximab combined with cisplatin and radiation therapy, was safely used in 45 patients with locally – advanced esophageal squamous cell cancer. Total-
ly 29 cases showed complete response and 15 showed partial response. But cetuximab plus irinotecan, cisplatin and radiation therapy
was toxic and did not achieve a better pCR rate in localized esophageal adenocarcinoma patients. In a clinical trial of patients with non –
metastatic esophageal cancer, the chemoradiotherapy (cisplatin,
capecitabine and radiotherapy) plus cetuximab treatment group had
fewer patients who were treatment failure free at 24 weeks, shorter
median overall survival and more non – haematological grade 3 or 4
toxicities than chemoradiotherapy treatment group, implying that the
addition of cetuximab to standard chemotherapy and radiotherapy
couldn't be recommended for esophageal cancer patients.

　　Panitumumab is a fully – humanized IgG2 mAb approved for the
treatment of metastatic colorectal cancer. It has considerably higher
binding affinity for EGFR, as compared with cetuximab. In a randomized, open – label clinical trial, the OS of patients with untreated,
metastatic or locally advanced esophagogastric adenocarcinoma wasn't
increased by the addition of panitumumab to epirubicin, oxaliplatin,
and capecitabine chemotherapy. The preoperative chemoradiotherapy
with docetaxel, cisplatin, and panitumumab was active in treating patients with locally advanced but resectable distal esophageal adenocarcinoma, but the toxicity was significant (48.5% had toxicity ⩾ grade
4). Another preoperative chemoradiotherapy regimen (panitumumab,

paclitaxel and radiation therapy) was safely received by esophageal adenocarcinoma patients with well tolerance, but it didn't improve pCR rate to the preset criterion of 40%.

Nimotuzumab has been intensively investigated in treating esophageal cancer. It was reported that nimotuzumab in combination with cisplatin/5 – FU regimen was safe and effective in patients with advanced esophageal squamous cell cancer. Furthermore, nimotuzumab in combination with irradiation or chemoradiation was safe and tolerable, and yielded encouraging OS (26. 0 months), PFS (16. 7 months) and two year locoregional control (80%). The combination of three – dimensional conformal radiotherapy and 200 mg nimotuzumab per week showed good therapeutic effects with 52. 4% PR, 40. 5% stable disease, 14 months median survival time, 10 months median PFS. Another clinical trial also showed that nimotuzumab combined with radiotherapy was safe and provided statistically significant objective response (47. 8%). Nimotuzumab enhanced the radiosensitivity of esophageal squamous cell cancer cells by upregulating IGFBP – 3. The esophageal squamous cell cancer patients with EGFR overexpression treated with nimotuzumab had higher objective response rate, but much shorter PFS and OS than those with low to moderate EGFR expression.

It has been reported that matuzumab in combination with PLF (high – dose 5 – fluorouracil, leucovorin and cisplatin) demonstrated an acceptable safety profile with modest anti – tumor activity in patients with advanced esophagogastric adenocarcinomas. But in a randomised, multicentre open – label study, the addition of matuzumab to ECX showed lower objective response, median PFS and median OS, and higher grade 3/4 toxicity rate in patients with metastatic esophagogastric cancer. Rao S. et al have found that the regimen of matuzumab and ECX could be well – tolerated and showed encouraging anti – tumour activity.

2.2 EGFRTKIs

The EGFRTKIs erlotinib, gefitinib have been approved to treat patients with metastatic non – small – cell lung cancer harbouring somatic mutations of the EGFR. It has been reported that gefitinib was well tolerated but of limited efficacy in recurrent or metastatic esophageal or gastroesophageal cancer patients. In another trial, the use of gefitinib as a second – line treatment in unselected esophageal cancer patients failed to improve the OS, but presented palliative benefits in some difficult – to – treat patients with short life expectancy. Gefitinib has also been found effective and tolerable in elderly patients with esophageal squamous cell cancer when combined with radiotherapy. When combined with chemoradiotherapy and surgery, gefitinib improved clinical outcomes in the definitive treatment of esophageal or gastroesophageal junction cancer.

Erlotinib has shown promising activity in different types of cancer, including pancreatic cancer as well as esophageal cancer. The patients with esophageal squamous cell cancer had longer time to tumor progression than those with esophageal adenocarcinoma when treated with 150 mg erlotinib daily, and the EGFR – positive cohort showed better response than the EGFR – negative cohort. mFOLFOX6 plus erlotinib was active and had an acceptable toxicity profile in patients with gastro – esophageal junction (GEJ) adenocarcinoma. The combined regimen of erlotinib and radiotherapy were tolerable and effective in chemoradiotherapy – intolerant esophageal squamous cell cancer patients. In one clinical study, erlotinib in combination with chemoradiotherapy presented satisfactory 2 – year OS and local – regional

control in patients with locally advanced esophageal cancer. But in another clinical trial, the patients with previously untreated localized e-
sophageal cancer didn't get survival benefit and improved pCR rate
from treatment with erlotinib and bevacizumab plus neoadjuvant chemoradiation (paclitaxel, carboplatin, 5 – FU and radiation therapy).

3. HER2 targeted therapy

HER2 is a transmembrane tyrosine kinase receptor that belongs to
EGFR family. HER2 overexpression may lead to transphoshorylation and
activation of downstream signaling pathways, including Ras – Raf –
MAPK and PI3K – AKT, which play oncogenic roles in various malignancies. HER2 amplification, positivity and overexpression are all
associated with poor cancer – specific survival of esophageal adenocarcinoma patients. HER2 amplification is observed in 11% (27/245)
of the esophageal squamous cell cancer specimens, and is a significant predictor of poor prognosis. HER2 overexpression is negatively
correlated with the development of esophageal cancer.

3. 1 Anti – HER2mAbs

The IgG1 mAb trastuzumab prevents heterodimerisation of HER2
receptor, triggers receptor internalisation and mediates antibody – dependent cellular cytotoxicity. Trastuzumab has been approved for the
adjuvant and palliative treatment of HER2 – positive breast cancer. It
has been reported that trastuzumab combined with chemotherapy was
effective and safe in HER2 – positive patients with advanced chemo –
refractory gastric or gastroesophageal junction adenocarninoma. Another trial showed that the regimen of modified FOLFOX6 plus trastuzumab was safe and efficient for patients with advanced gastroesophageal
junction cancer. Trastuzumab – based therapy was also active in combination with several other chemotherapeutic regimens in advanced

esophagogastric cance.

3. 2 Anti – HER2TKIs

Lapatinib, a dual TKI which simultaneously inhibits EGFR and HER2, has been approved for the treatment of patients with metastatic HER2 – positive breast cancer. Recently, several clinical trials have evaluated the efficacy and safety of lapatinib in esophageal cancer. The combination of lapatinib and 5 – fluorouracil or cisplatin can synergistically inhibit the proliferation and can promote the apoptosis of esophageal cancer cells through inhibiting the phosphorylation of EGFR and HER2. Lapatinib can also inhibit the growth of esophageal squamous cell cancer and synergistically interact with 5 – fluorouracil in patient – derived xenograft models. The addition of lapatinib to capecitabine and oxaliplatin in the first – line treatment of patients with HER2 – positive gastric cancer can't lead to prolonged OS. Esophageal squamous cell cancer patients with overexpressed HER2 are considered as good candidates for the HER2 targeted therapy, and the combination of Herceptin and lapatinib is a new promising strategy for HER2 positive esophageal squamous cell cancer patients.

4. VEGFR targeted therapy

VEGF is the most potentproangiogenic factor that interacts with VEGFRs. VEGF – mediated angiogenesis may play important roles in the development of esophageal cancer. VEGFR expression was observed in 53.8% (77/154) esophageal adenocarcinoma patients and was correlated with poor survival.

4. 1 Anti – VEGF/VEGFRmAbs

Bevacizumab is a recombinant humanized mAb (IgG1) targeting VEGF and has been approved for treatment of metastatic colorectal, ovarian, breast, renal cell and non – small – cell lung cancer. In several clinical studies of patients with metastatic esophagogastric adenocarcinoma, bevacizumab in combination with chemotherapy, for example, capecitabine plus oxaliplatin, cisplatin plus 5 – FU, ECX or mDCF, was proved to be active and well tolerated. However, the addition of bevacizumab and erlotinib to neoadjuvant chemoradiotherapy (paclitaxel, carboplatin, 5 – FU and radiation) did not show survival benefit.

Ramucirumab is another fully humanized mAb that binds to VEGFR2. In an international, randomised, multicentre, placebo – controlled clinical trial, 355 enrolled patients with advanced gastric or GEJ adenocarcinoma and disease progression after first – line chemotherapy were randomly assigned to receive ramucirumab or placebo therapy, and the patients in the ramucirumab group got longer median OS. Another clinical trial of patients with previously treated advanced gastric or gastro – esophageal junction adenocarcinoma showed that the OS was significantly longer in the ramucirumab group than in the placebo group. Taken together, bevacizumab and ramucirumab have shown good activity and well tolerance in esophageal cancer therapy.

4.2 Anti – VEGFRTKIs

Sorafenib is a broad spectrum TKI that targets VEGFR2, and has been approved for the treatment of renal cell carcinoma and hepatocellular carcinoma. In the chemotherapy refractory patients with metastatic esophageal and GEJ cancer, sorafenib treatment results in disease stabilization and encouraging PFS, but with uncommon grade 3 toxicities of hand foot skin reaction, rash, dehydration and fatigue.

Sunitinib is an oral small molecule multi – targeted TKI and has been approved for the treatment of advanced renal cell carcinoma and imatinib resistant or intolerant gastrointestinal stromal tumors. In a single – stage clinical study, sunitinib is well tolerated in the 25 enrolled patients with relapsed/refractory esophageal and gastroesophageal cancers. Another clinical study showed that the patients with advanced esophageal or gastroesophageal junction cancer in the sunitinib plus paclitaxel group received a no better 24 – week PFS and a higher rate of serious toxicities than that in historical controls.

Pazopanib is an oral agent which prevents angiogenesis through inhibiting the VEGFR, PDGFR and c – Kit. It has been approved for the treatment of metastatic renal cell carcinoma as well as metastatic soft tissue sarcoma. In a multicenter, open – label clinical study, the patients with advanced solid tumors were treated with paclitaxel in combination with carboplatin and daily pazopanib. As a result, two patients with esophageal cancer got complete response, and one patient with gastroesophageal junction cancer had partial response.

5. c – MET targeted therapy

c – MET is widely expressed in cells of epithelial – endothelial origin. c – MET is overexpressed in many cancers, including lung, breast, ovary, kidney, colon, thyroid, liver, and gastric cancers. To date, many agents have developed to target c – MET, such as rilotumumab, tivantinib, cabozantinib, foretinib, crizotinib and PHA665752.

5. 1 Anti – c – METmAbs

Rilotumumab is a mAb that interferes with c – MET's activation and decreases c – MET phosphorylation. In an open – label, dose de – escalation study and a double – blind, randomized clinical study, rilotumumab plus ECX showed greater activity than placebo plus ECX in patients with unresectable locally advanced or metastatic gastric or GEJ adenocarcinoma. However, the adverse events were more common in the rilotumumab group than in the placebo group. More clinical trials should be performed to evaluate the efficacy and safety of rilotumumab in patients with advanced esophageal cancer, alone or in combination with chemotherapy or radiotherapy.

5. 2 Anti – c – MET inhibitors

PHA665752 can selectively inhibits c – MET in tumor cells, leading to arrested cell cycle, decreased motility and migration and increased apoptosis. Activity of this drug can be enhanced by concurrent use of rapamycin. PHA665752 can inhibit the tumorigenicity and angiogenesis in mouse lung cancer xenograft. The effect of PHA665752 on cell viability, apoptosis, motility, invasion has been studied in three c – MET – overexpressing esophageal adenocarcinoma cell lines. The results showed that PHA665752 inhibited the cell viability, motility and invasion and induced cell apoptosis. Taken together, c – MET inhibition may be a useful therapeutic strategy for esophageal adenocarcinoma.

6. Expert commentary

The prognosis of patients with advanced esophageal cancer is very poor due to lack of effective therapeutic agents. So far, a variety of molecular targeted agents have been developed, alone or in combination with chemotherapy, radiotherapy orchemoradiotherapy, to improve the outcomes of esophageal cancer (Table 1).

Table 1　mAbs and TKIs in phase II/III trials for advanced esophageal or esophagogastric cancer

Agent	Phase	N	Treatmen Regimen	Median OS	Median PFS	
Cetuximab	II	150	DOCOX ± cetuximab	8.5 months vs 9.4 months	4.7 months vs 5.1 months	
Cetuximab	II	19	irinotecan + cisplatin + radiotherapy + cetuximab	31 months	10 months	*
Cetuximab	II/III	258	cisplatin + capecitabine + radiotherapy ± cetuximab	22.1 months vs 25.4 months	–	*
Panitumumab	III	553	mEOC ± panitumumab	8.8 months vs 11.3 months	–	*
Panitumumab	II	70	DCP + radiotherapy	19.4 months	–	**
Nimotuzumab	–	66	chemoradiotherapy/radiotherapy + nimotuzumab	26.0 months	16.7 months	**
Matuzumab	II	72	ECX ± matuzumab	9.4 months vs 12.2 months	4.8 months vs 7.1 months	*
Gefitinib	II	58	gefitinib	5.5 months	–	
Gefitinib	II	20	radiotherapy + gefitinib	14.0 months	7.0 months	**
Erlotinib	II	33	mFOLFOX6 + erlotinib	11.0 months	5.5 months	*
Erlotinib	–	18	radiotherapy + erlotinib	21.1 months	12 months	**
Erlotinib	II	17	radiotherapy + erlotinib	7.3 months	4.5 months	**
Trastuzumab	–	20	chemotherapy + trastuzumab	11.1 months	6.1 months	*
Trastuzumab	–	34	mFOLFOX6/ XELOX + trastuzumab	17.3 months	9.0 months	*
Bevacizumab	II	44	mDCF + bevacizumab	16.8 months	12 months	*
Bevacizumab	II	37	capecitabine + oxaliplatin + bevacizumab	10.8 months	7.2 months	*
Ramucirumab	II	355	ramucirumab vs placebo	5.2 months vs 3.8 months	–	
Ramucirumab	II	665	ramucirumab + paclitaxel vs placebo + paclitaxel	9.6 months vs 7.4 months	–	
Sorafenib	II	34	sorafenib	9.7 months	3.6 months	
Sunitinib	II	25	sunitinib	17 weeks	7 weeks	
Sunitinib	II	28	paclitaxel + sunitinib	228 days	–	
Rilotumumab	II	121	ECX + rilotumumab (15mg/kg) vs ECX + rilotumumab(7.5mg/kg) vs ECX + placebo	–	5.1 months vs 6.8 months vs 4.2 months	

N: number; DOCOX: docetaxel, cetuximab and oxaliplatin; m: modified; EOC: epirubicin, oxaliplatin, and capecitabine; DCP: docetaxel, cisplatin, and panitumumab; ECX: epirubicin, cisplatin, and capecitabine; FOLFOX6: oxaliplatin, fluorouracil and leucovorin; XELOX: capecitabine and oxaliplatin; DCF: docetaxel, cisplatin, and fluorouracil; ECX: epirubicin, cisplatin, and capecitabine; OS: overall survival; PFS: progression – free survival. *, the references relating to esophageal adenocarcinoma; **, the references for esophageal squamous cell carcinoma.

As shown in Figure 1, EGFR, HER2, VEGR and c – MET are known as valuable targets for esophageal cancer. The inhibitors of these targets have shown efficacy with or without intolerable toxicities. The molecular targeted therapy may lead to acquired resistance. Dysregulation of EGFR internalization and degradation, and genetic mutations in RAS, RAF, AKT and PI3K may lead to resistance to EGFR antibody. Genetic alterations in the PI3K/AKT pathway are correlated with resistance to HER2 – targeted therapy. Resistance to antiangiogenic therapy may be due to several mechanisms, including differentiation of cancer stem cells into endothelial cells, development of cytogenetic abnormalities in tumor endothelial cells, and recruiting of tumor vessels via VEGF – independent pathways. The mechanisms of resistance to c – MET targeted agents involve up – regulation of HER kinase signaling, mutation of the MET activation loop and amplification of KRAS.

Although the function of EGFR, HER2, VEGR and c – MET is widely studied, the exact molecular mechanism of these targets in esophageal cancer are unclear. Continued basic research on the mechanism of these targets may lead to novel diagnostic and therapeutic approaches. There is much to be learned concerning the mechanisms of these targets that contribute to chemoresistance in esophageal cancer.

Some clinical trials have to be stopped because of serious adverse events. Thus, it is needed to investigate whether the correct therapeutic outcome is achieved without any unanticipated side effects. Various approaches combining different agents with existing and novel treatment modalities will continue to be explored to maximize therapeutic benefits. Further research are required to identify reliable and predictive biomarkers that assist in selecting patients who are likely to benefit from targeted therapy with minimal toxicities. Analysis of SNPs and whole exome/transcriptome sequencing will help to identify the right patient population in the era of personalized medicine.

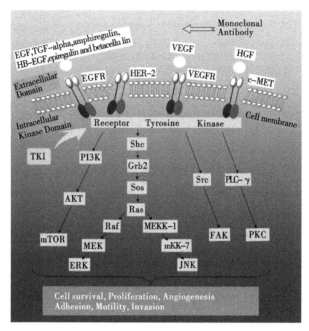

Figure 1　EGFR, HER – 2, VEGFR and c – MET related signal pathways. EGFR, HER – 2, VEGFR and c – MET are activated by ligand binding to extracellular domain, then leading to auto – phosphorylation of intracellular tyrosine residues. Intracellular signaling pathways involve PI3K/AKT/mTOR, Ras/Raf/MEK/ERK, Ras/MEKK – 1/MKK – 7/JNK, Src/FAK and PLC – γ/PKC

7. Five – year view

During recent years, the molecular targeted therapy has been developing as a promising effective treatment in esophageal cancer. Although most of the molecular targeted agents are still under stages of clinical trials, some have showed their advantages in cancer therapy.

More research will focus on clarifying the pathogenesis of esophageal cancer, searching more effective and less toxic regimens, and identifying result evaluation systems. With the advancement of scientific and technological methods, we would see significant progress in understanding of the effective molecular targeted therapy in the near future.

Key issues

1. The incidence of esophageal cancer is increasing, and the prognosis is poor due to lack of effective therapy.

2. EGFR, HER – 2, VEGFR and c – MET – play important roles in the proliferation, differentiation, invasion, angiogenesis and apoptosis of esophageal cancer cells.

3. The results of many clinical trials have shown that EGFR, HER2, VEGR and c – MET are valuable therapeutic targets for esophageal cancer.

4. Continued basic research on the mechanism of EGFR, HER2, VEGR and c – MET in esophageal cancer may lead to novel diagnostic and therapeutic approaches.

5. More clinical trials should be performed to evaluate the benefits of combiningtargeted therapy with chemotherapy and radiotherapy basing on a patient's molecular profile.

Acknowledgement

This study was supported in part by grants from the National Natural Scientific Foundation of China (81171923). There is no conflict of interest.

（张　磊　马娇娇　韩　宇　柳金强　周　威　洪　流　樊代明）

References

[1] Pennathur A, Gibson MK, Jobe BA, et al. Oesophageal carcinoma. LANCET,2013,381:400 – 412.

[2] Torre LA, Bray F, Siegel RL, et al. Global cancer statistics,2012. CA Cancer J Clin,2015,65:87 – 108.

[3] Smithers BM, Gotley DC, Martin I, et al. Comparison of the outcomes between open and minimally invasive esophagectomy. ANN SURG, 2007, 245:232 – 240.

[4] Birkmeyer JD, Siewers AE, Finlayson EV, et al. Hospital volume and surgical mortality in the United States. N Engl J Med,2002,346:1128 – 1137.

[5] Cappetta A, Lonardi S, Pastorelli D, et al. Advanced gastric cancer (GC) and cancer of the gastro – oesophageal junction (GEJ): focus on targeted therapies. Crit Rev Oncol Hematol,2012,81:38 – 48.

[6] Enzinger PC, Mayer RJ. Esophageal cancer. N Engl J Med, 2003, 349: 2241 – 2252.

[7] Ajani JA, Moiseyenko VM, Tjulandin S, et al. Clinical benefit with docetaxel plus fluorouracil and cisplatin compared with cisplatin and fluorouracil in a phase Ⅲ trial of advanced gastric or gastroesophageal cancer adenocarcinoma: the V – 325 Study Group. J CLIN ONCOL,2007,25: 3205 – 3209.

[8] Van Cutsem E, Moiseyenko VM, Tjulandin S, et al. Phase Ⅲ study of docetaxel and cisplatin plus fluorouracil compared with cisplatin and fluorouracil as first – line therapy for advanced gastric cancer: a report of the V325 Study Group. J CLIN ONCOL,2006,24:4991 – 4997.

[9] Ferguson KM. Structure – based view of epidermal growth factor receptor regulation. ANNU REV BIOPHYS,2008,37:353 – 373.

[10] Ayyappan S, Prabhakar D, Sharma N. Epidermal growth factor receptor

（EGFR）- targeted therapies in esophagogastric cancer. ANTICANCER RES,2013,33:4139 -4155.

[11] Norguet E, Dahan L, Seitz JF. Targetting esophageal and gastric cancers with monoclonal antibodies. CURR TOP MED CHEM,2012,12:1678 - 1682.

[12] Liang J, E M, Wu G, et al. Nimotuzumab combined with radiotherapy for e-sophageal cancer: preliminary study of a Phase Ⅱ clinical trial. Onco Targets Ther,2013,6:1589 - 1596.

[13] Wang J, Yu JM, Jing SW, et al. Relationship between EGFR over - expression and clinicopathologic characteristics in squamous cell carcinoma of the esophagus: a meta - analysis. Asian Pac J Cancer Prev,2014,15: 5889 - 5893.

[14] Li JC, Zhao YH, Wang XY, et al. Clinical significance of the expression of EGFR signaling pathway - related proteins in esophageal squamous cell carcinoma. Tumour Biol,2014,35:651 - 657.

[15] Jiang D, Li X, Wang H, et al. The prognostic value of EGFR overexpression and amplification in Esophageal squamous cell Carcinoma. BMC CANCER,2015,15:377.

[16] Goldstein NI, Prewett M, Zuklys K,et al. Biological efficacy of a chimeric antibody to the epidermal growth factor receptor in a human tumor xenograft model. CLIN CANCER RES,1995,1:1311 - 1318.

[17] Kasper S, Schuler M. Targeted therapies in gastroesophageal cancer. EUR J CANCER,2014,50:1247 - 1258.

[18] Miller JA, Ford DJ, Ahmed MS, et al. Two Cases of Pneumatosis Intestinalis during Cetuximab Therapy for Advanced Head and Neck Cancer. Case Rep Oncol Med,2015,2015:214 - 236.

[19] Kurokawa M, Watanabe NM, Harada R, et al. Initial experience of radiotherapy plus cetuximab for Japanese head and neck cancer patients. J RADIAT RES,2015,56:849 - 855.

[20] Liu D, Zheng X, Chen J, et al. Induction chemotherapy with cetuximab, vinorelbine - cisplatin followed by thoracic radiotherapy and concurrent cetuximab, vinorelbine - cisplatin in patients with unresectable stage Ⅲ

non – small cell lung cancer. LUNG CANCER,2015,89:249 – 254.

[21] Vansteenkiste J, Barlesi F, Waller CF, et al. Cilengitide combined with cetuximab and platinum – based chemotherapy as first – line treatment in advanced non – small – cell lung cancer (NSCLC) patients: results of an open – label, randomized, controlled phase Ⅱ study (CERTO). ANN ONCOL,2015,26:1734 – 1740.

[22] Tian J, Shang M, Shi SB, et al. Cetuximab plus pemetrexed as second – line therapy for fluorouracil – based pre – treated metastatic esophageal squamous cell carcinoma. Cancer Chemother Pharmacol,2015,76:829 – 834.

[23] Utsunomiya S, Uehara K, Kurimoto T, et al. Synchronous rectal and esophageal cancer treated with chemotherapy followed by two – stage resec tion. World J Clin Cases,2013,1:87 – 91.

[24] Tebbutt NC, Parry MM, Zannino D, et al. Docetaxel plus cetuximab as second – line treatment for docetaxel – refractory oesophagogastric cancer: the AGITG ATTAX2 trial. Br J Cancer,2013,108:771 – 774.

[25] Ubink I, van der Sluis P, Schipper M, et al. Adding preoperative radiotherapy plus cetuximab to perioperative chemotherapy for resectable esophageal adenocarcinoma: a single – center prospective phaseⅡtrial. ONCOLOGIST, 2014,19:32 – 33.

[26] Becerra CR, Hanna N, McCollum AD, et al. A phase II study with cetuximab and radiation therapy for patients with surgically resectable esophageal and GE junction carcinomas: Hoosier Oncology Group G05 – 92. J THORAC ONCOL,2013,8:1425 – 1429.

[27] Richards D, Kocs DM, Spira AI, et al. Results of docetaxel plus oxaliplatin (DOCOX) + / – cetuximab in patients with metastatic gastric and/or gastroesophageal junction adenocarcinoma: results of a randomised Phase 2 study. EUR J CANCER,2013,49:2823 – 2831.

[28] Meng X, Wang J, Sun X, et al. Cetuximab in combination with chemoradiotherapy in Chinese patients with non – resectable, locally advanced esophageal squamous cell carcinoma: a prospective, multicenter phase Ⅱ trail. RADIOTHER ONCOL,2013,109:275 – 280.

[29] Lee MS, Mamon HJ, Hong TS, et al. Preoperative cetuximab, irinotecan, cisplatin, and radiation therapy for patients with locally advanced esophageal cancer. ONCOLOGIST,2013,18:281 - 287.

[30] Crosby T, Hurt CN, Falk S, et al. Chemoradiotherapy with or without cetuximab in patients with oesophageal cancer (SCOPE1): a multicentre, phase 2/3 randomised trial. LANCET ONCOL,2013,14:627 - 637.

[31] Grothey A. EGFR antibodies in colorectal cancer: where do they belong. J CLIN ONCOL,2010,28:4668 - 4670.

[32] Sliwkowski MX, Mellman I. Antibody therapeutics in cancer. SCIENCE 2013,341:1192 - 1198.

[33] Okines AF, Gonzalez DCD, Cunningham D, et al. Biomarker analysis in oesophagogastric cancer: Results from the REAL3 and TransMAGIC trials. EUR J CANCER,2013,49:2116 - 2125.

[34] Lockhart AC, Reed CE, Decker PA, et al. Phase Ⅱ study of neoadjuvant therapy with docetaxel, cisplatin, panitumumab, and radiation therapy followed by surgery in patients with locally advanced adenocarcinoma of the distal esophagus (ACOSOG Z4051). ANN ONCOL,2014,25:1039 - 1044.

[35] Kordes S, van Berge HM, Hulshof MC, et al. Preoperative chemoradiation therapy in combination with panitumumab for patients with resectable esophageal cancer: the PACT study. Int J Radiat Oncol Biol Phys, 2014,90:190 - 196.

[36] Ling Y, Chen J, Tao M, et al. A pilot study of nimotuzumab combined with cisplatin and 5 - FU in patients with advanced esophageal squamous cell carcinoma. J Thorac Dis,2012,4:58 - 62.

[37] Ma NY, Cai XW, Fu XL, et al. Safety and efficacy of nimotuzumab in combination with radiotherapy for patients with squamous cell carcinoma of the esophagus. INT J CLIN ONCOL,2014,19:297 - 302.

[38] Liang J, E M, Wu G, et al. Nimotuzumab combined with radiotherapy for esophageal cancer: preliminary study of a Phase Ⅱ clinical trial. Onco Targets Ther,2013,6:1589 - 1596.

[39] Ramos - Suzarte M, Lorenzo - Luaces P, Lazo NG, et al. Treatment of malig-

nant, non – resectable, epithelial origin esophageal tumours with the humanized anti – epidermal growth factor antibody nimotuzumab combined with radiation therapy and chemotherapy. CANCER BIOL THER, 2012, 13:
600 – 605.

[40] Zhao L, He LR, Xi M, et al. Nimotuzumab promotes radiosensitivity of
EGFR – overexpression esophageal squamous cell carcinoma cells by upregulating IGFBP – 3. J TRANSL MED,2012,10:249.

[41] Jia J, Cui Y, Lu M, et al. The relation of EGFR expression by immunohistochemical staining and clinical response of combination treatment of
nimotuzumab and chemotherapy in esophageal squamous cell carcinoma.
CLIN TRANSL ONCOL,2015,18(6):592 – 598.

[42] Trarbach T, Przyborek M, Schleucher N, et al. Phase I study of matuzumab in combination with 5 – fluorouracil, leucovorin and cisplatin
(PLF) in patients with advanced gastric and esophagogastric adenocarcinomas. Invest New Drugs,2013,31:642 – 652.

[43] Rao S, Starling N, Cunningham D, et al. Matuzumab plus epirubicin,
cisplatin and capecitabine (ECX) compared with epirubicin, cisplatin
and capecitabine alone as first – line treatment in patients with advanced
oesophago – gastric cancer: a randomised, multicentre open – label phase
II study. ANN ONCOL,2010,21:2213 – 2219.

[44] Rao S, Starling N, Cunningham D, et al. Phase I study of epirubicin,
cisplatin and capecitabine plus matuzumab in previously untreated patients with advanced oesophagogastric cancer. Br J Cancer, 2008, 99:
868 – 874.

[45] Adelstein DJ, Rodriguez CP, Rybicki LA, et al. A phase II trial of gefitinib for recurrent or metastatic cancer of the esophagus or gastroesophageal junction. Invest New Drugs 2012;30:1684 – 1689.

[46] Xu Y, Zheng Y, Sun X, et al. Concurrent radiotherapy with gefitinib in
elderly patients with esophageal squamous cell carcinoma: Preliminary results of a phase II study. ONCOTARGET,2015,6(35):38429 – 38439.

[47] Sohal DP, Rice TW, Rybicki LA, et al. Gefitinib in definitive manage-

ment of esophageal or gastroesophageal junction cancer: a retrospective a-nalysis of two clinical trials. DIS ESOPHAGUS,2015,28:547 – 551.

[48] Kris MG, Natale RB, Herbst RS, et al. Efficacy of gefitinib, an inhibitor of the epidermal growth factor receptor tyrosine kinase, in symptomatic patients with non – small cell lung cancer: a randomized trial. JAMA, 2003,290:2149 – 2158.

[49] Ilson DH, Kelsen D, Shah M, et al. A phase 2 trial of erlotinib in pa-tients with previously treated squamous cell and adenocarcinoma of the e-sophagus. CANCER – AM CANCER SOC,2011,117:1409 – 1414.

[50] Wainberg ZA, Lin LS, DiCarlo B, et al. Phase Ⅱ trial of modified FOL-FOX6 and erlotinib in patients with metastatic or advanced adenocarcino-ma of the oesophagus and gastro – oesophageal junction. Br J Cancer, 2011,105:760 – 765.

[51] Zhai Y, Hui Z, Wang J, et al. Concurrent erlotinib and radiotherapy for chemoradiotherapy – intolerant esophageal squamous cell carcinoma pa-tients: results of a pilot study. DIS ESOPHAGUS,2013,26:503 – 509.

[52] Zhang XB, Xie CY, Li WF, et al. Phase II study of radiotherapy plus er-lotinib for elder patients with esophageal carcinoma. Zhonghua Yi Xue Za Zhi,2012,92:1615 – 1617.

[53] Iyer R, Chhatrala R, Shefter T, et al. Erlotinib and radiation therapy for elderly patients with esophageal cancer – clinical and correlative results from a prospective multicenter phase 2 trial. ONCOLOGY – BASEL, 2013,85:53 – 58.

[54] Li G, Hu W, Wang J, et al. Phase Ⅱ study of concurrent chemoradiation in combination with erlotinib for locally advanced esophageal carcinoma. Int J Radiat Oncol Biol Phys,2010,78:1407 – 1412.

[55] Bendell JC, Meluch A, Peyton J, et al. A phase Ⅱ trial of preoperative concurrent chemotherapy/radiation therapy plus bevacizumab/erlotinib in the treatment of localized esophageal cancer. Clin Adv Hematol Oncol 2012,10:430 – 437.

[56] Thiel A, Ristimaki A. Targeted therapy in gastric cancer. APMIS,2015,

123：365 - 372.

[57] Prins MJ, Ruurda JP, van Diest PJ, et al. The significance of the HER - 2 status in esophageal adenocarcinoma for survival: an immunohistochemical and an in situ hybridization study. ANN ONCOL,2013,24:1290 - 1297.

[58] Kato H, Arao T, Matsumoto K, et al. Gene amplification of EGFR, HER2, FGFR2 and MET in esophageal squamous cell carcinoma. INT J ONCOL,2013,42:1151 - 1158.

[59] Gonzaga IM, Soares - Lima SC, de Santos PT, et al. Alterations in epidermal growth factor receptors 1 and 2 in esophageal squamous cell carcinomas. BMC CANCER,2012,12:569.

[60] Zhang X, Wu Y, Gong J, et al. Trastuzumab combined with chemotherapy in patients with HER2 - positive chemo - refractory advanced gastric or gastro - esophageal junction adenocarcinoma. Zhonghua Zhong Liu Za Zhi,2014,36:223 - 227.

[61] Soularue E, Cohen R, Tournigand C, et al. Efficacy and safety of trastuzumab in combination with oxaliplatin and fluorouracil - based chemotherapy for patients with HER2 - positive metastatic gastric and gastro - oesophageal junction adenocarcinoma patients: a retrospective study. Bull Cancer,2015,102:324 - 331.

[62] Haag GM, Apostolidis L, Jaeger D. Efficacy and safety of trastuzumab - based therapy in combination with different chemotherapeutic regimens in advanced esophagogastric cancer—a single cancer - center experience. TUMORI,2014,100:237 - 242.

[63] Guo XF, Zhu XF, Zhong GS, et al. Lapatinib, a dual inhibitor of EGFR and HER2, has synergistic effects with 5 - fluorouracil on esophageal carcinoma. ONCOL REP,2012,27:1639 - 1645.

[64] Guo XF, Zhu XF, Zhong GS, et al. Lapatinib, a dual inhibitor of epidermal growth factor receptor and human epidermal growth factor receptor 2, potentiates the antitumor effects of cisplatin on esophageal carcinoma. DIS ESOPHAGUS,2013,26:487 - 495.

[65] Mimura K, Izawa S, Siba S, et al. The effect of immune - based therapy

with cytotoxic T lymphocyte and molecular targeting therapy for HER2 in esophageal squamous cell carcinoma. Gan To Kagaku Ryoho, 2011, 38: 1918 – 1920.

[66] Prins MJ, Verhage RJ, Ten KF, et al. Cyclooxygenase isoenzyme – 2 and vascular endothelial growth factor are associated with poor prognosis in e-sophageal adenocarcinoma. J GASTROINTEST SURG, 2012, 16:956 – 966.

[67] Okines AF, Langley RE, Thompson LC, et al. Bevacizumab with peri – operative epirubicin, cisplatin and capecitabine (ECX) in localised gastro – oesophageal adenocarcinoma: a safety report. ANN ONCOL, 2013, 24:702 – 709.

[68] Shah MA, Jhawer M, Ilson DH, et al. Phase II study of modified docetaxel, cisplatin, and fluorouracil with bevacizumab in patients with metastatic gastroesophageal adenocarcinoma. J CLIN ONCOL, 2011, 29:868 – 874.

[69] Uronis HE, Bendell JC, Altomare I, et al. A phase II study of capecitabine, oxaliplatin, and bevacizumab in the treatment of metastatic esophagogastric adenocarcinomas. ONCOLOGIST, 2013, 18:271 – 272.

[70] Bendell JC, Meluch A, Peyton J, et al. A phase II trial of preoperative concurrent chemotherapy/radiation therapy plus bevacizumab/erlotinib in the treatment of localized esophageal cancer. Clin Adv Hematol Oncol, 2012, 10:430 – 437.

[71] Fuchs CS, Tomasek J, Yong CJ, et al. Ramucirumab monotherapy for previously treated advanced gastric or gastro – oesophageal junction adenocarcinoma (REGARD): an international, randomised, multicentre, placebo – controlled, phase 3 trial. LANCET, 2014, 383:31 – 39.

[72] Wilke H, Muro K, Van Cutsem E, et al. Ramucirumab plus paclitaxel versus placebo plus paclitaxel in patients with previously treated advanced gastric or gastro – oesophageal junction adenocarcinoma (RAINBOW): a double – blind, randomised phase 3 trial. LANCET ONCOL, 2014, 15:1224 – 1235.

[73] Escudier B, Eisen T, Stadler WM, et al. Sorafenib in advanced clear – cell renal – cell carcinoma. N Engl J Med, 2007, 356:125 – 134.

[74] Llovet JM, Ricci S, Mazzaferro V, et al. Sorafenib in advanced hepato-

cellular carcinoma. N Engl J Med,2008,359:378 - 390.

[75] Janjigian YY, Vakiani E, Ku GY, et al. Phase Ⅱ Trial of Sorafenib in Patients with Chemotherapy Refractory Metastatic Esophageal and Gastroesophageal (GE) Junction Cancer. PLOS ONE,2015,10:e134731.

[76] Wu C, Mikhail S, Wei L, et al. A phase Ⅱ and pharmacodynamic study of sunitinib in relapsed/refractory oesophageal and gastro - oesophageal cancers. Br J Cancer,2015,113:220 - 225.

[77] Schmitt JM, Sommers SR, Fisher W, et al. Sunitinib plus paclitaxel in patients with advanced esophageal cancer: a phase Ⅱ study from the Hoosier Oncology Group. J THORAC ONCOL,2012,7:760 - 763.

[78] Burris HR, Dowlati A, Moss RA, et al. Phase I study of pazopanib in combination with paclitaxel and carboplatin given every 21 days in patients with advanced solid tumors. MOL CANCER THER,2012,11:1820 - 1828.

[79] van der Graaf WT, Blay JY, Chawla SP, et al. Pazopanib for metastatic soft - tissue sarcoma (PALETTE): a randomised, double - blind, placebo - controlled phase 3 trial. LANCET,2012,379:1879 - 1886.

[80] Sternberg CN, Davis ID, Mardiak J, et al. Pazopanib in locally advanced or metastatic renal cell carcinoma: results of a randomized phase Ⅲ trial. J CLIN ONCOL,2010,28:1061 - 1068.

[81] Bible KC, Suman VJ, Molina JR, et al. Efficacy of pazopanib in progressive, radioiodine - refractory, metastatic differentiated thyroid cancers: results of a phase 2 consortium study. LANCET ONCOL,2010,11:962 -972.

[82] Sierra JR, Tsao MS. c - MET as a potential therapeutic target and biomarker in cancer. Ther Adv Med Oncol,2011,3:S21 - S35.

[83] Iveson T, Donehower RC, Davidenko I, et al. Rilotumumab in combination with epirubicin, cisplatin, and capecitabine as first - line treatment for gastric or oesophagogastric junction adenocarcinoma: an open - label, dose de - escalation phase 1b study and a double - blind, randomised phase 2 study. LANCET ONCOL,2014,15:1007 - 1018.

[84] Lawrence RE, Salgia R. MET molecular mechanisms and therapies in

lung cancer. Cell Adh Migr,2010,4:146 – 152.

[85] Puri N, Khramtsov A, Ahmed S, et al. A selective small molecule inhibitor of c – Met, PHA665752, inhibits tumorigenicity and angiogenesis in mouse lung cancer xenografts. CANCER RES,2007,67:3529 – 3534.

[86] Watson GA, Zhang X, Stang MT, et al. Inhibition of c – Met as a therapeutic strategy for esophageal adenocarcinoma. NEOPLASIA,2006,8:949 – 955.

[87] Aprile G, Ongaro E, Del Re M, et al. Angiogenic inhibitors in gastric cancers and gastroesophageal junction carcinomas: A critical insight. Crit Rev Oncol Hematol,2015,95:165 – 78.

[88] Qi J, McTigue MA, Rogers A, et al. Multiple Mutations and Bypass Mechanisms Can Contribute to Development of Acquired Resistance to MET Inhibitors. Cancer Research,2011,71:1081 – 1091.

[89] Cepero V, Sierra JR, Corso S, et al. MET and KRAS Gene Amplification Mediates Acquired Resistance to MET Tyrosine Kinase Inhibitors. Cancer Research,2010,70:7580 – 7590.

（原文发表于 Expert Rev Gastroenterol Hepatol,2016,10:595 – 604）

综述二

Epigenetic roles in the malignant transformation of gastric mucosal cells

Abstract

Gastric carcinogenesis occurs when gastric epithelial cells transition through the initial, immortal, premalignant and malignant stages of transformation. Epigenetic regulations contributes to this multi – step process. Due to the critical role of epigenetic modifications, these changes are highly likely to be of clinical use in the future as new biomarkers and therapeutic targets for the early detection and treatment of cancers. Here, we summarize the recent findings on how epigenetic modifications, including DNA methylation, histone modifications and non – coding RNAs, regulate gastric carcinogenesis, and we discuss potential new strategies for the diagnosis and treatments of gastric cancer. The strategies may be helpful in the further understanding of epigenetic regulation in human diseases.

Key words: Epigenetic roles, Malignant transformation, Gastric mucosal cells, Helicobacter pylori

Introduction

The latest figures from the World Health Organization (WHO) show that 951 600 new gastric cancer cases and 723 100 gastric cancer – related deaths occurred globally in 2012. The overall incidence of gastric cancer has declined. However, in China, the morbidity and mortality of gastric cancer rank 2nd and 3rd, respectively, among all malignant tumors. Gastric cancer is classified into the following two subtypes: diffuse and intestinal. Usually, intestinal gastric cancers retain a glandular structure, and undergoe multiple processes, as follows: chronic inflammation, atrophy, intestinal metaplasia and atypical hyperplasia and eventually into gastric cancer. However, diffuse gastric cancer is relatively rare and is poorly differentiated to the extent that no glandular structure is recognizable. At present, no clear precancerous lesions of diffuse gastric cancer have been defined. Helicobacter pylori (H. pylori) infection plays an important carcinogenic role in both subtypes of gastric cancer. Many trials have demonstrated the possibility of cancer prevention through H. pylori screening and eradication. The malignant transformation of gastric mucosa involves multimolecular events including gene mutation and epigenetic alteration. This article presents a review of the roles of epigenetic alterations in the malignant transformation of gastric mucosa.

The concept and significance of epigenetics

The concept of epigenetics was first proposed by Waddington in 1939. Epigenetics refers to the heritable changes in gene expression that are independent of variations in DNA sequences. The main types of epigenetic processes include DNA methylation, histone modification, and chromatin remodeling as well as the function of non – coding RNA (ncRNA). The basic theory of classical genetics cannot adequately explain the biodiversity within species. For example, identical twins carrying the same DNA sequences may exhibit distinct phenotypes and different susceptibility to diseases. The proposal of epigenetics has compensated for such shortcoming of classical genetic theory. Epigenetics is a component of normal physiological regulation, and abnormal epigenetic regulation may lead to tumorigenesis. Studies have suggested that intestinal – type gastric cancer originates from chronic gastritis, which gradually progresses through stages of chronic atrophic gastritis, intestinal metaplasia and atypical hyperplasia and ultimately develops into advanced gastric cancer. During the malignant transformation of gastric mucosa, a large number of genes are subjected to epigenetic regulation. The genes show cumulative changes as the disease evolves.

Methylation of tumor suppressor genes is an important mechanism responsible for malignant transformation of gastric mucosa

Methylation is a type of chemical modification that occurs in DNA sequences. In mammalian cells, DNA methylation occurs almost exclusively at the fifth carbon atom of the cytosine residues within cytosine – phosphate – guanine (CpG) dinucleotides. CpG dinucleotides tend to form CG – rich clusters called CpG islands. CpG islands are mainly distributed in the core promoter sequence and transcription start site of structural genes. DNA methylation may induce changes in chromatin structure, DNA conformation, DNA stability and the interactions between DNA and protein, resulting in transcription inhibition. Two adverse phenomena characterize the process of carcinogenesis: locus – specific hypermethylation and global depletion of methyl groups from cancer genomes. Hypermethylation of promoters has been widely shown to contribute to the silencing of tumor suppressor genes during carcinogenesis. Global hypomethylation of the cancer genome was initially shown to cause genome – wide allelic instability, but recently, the involvement of this process in transcriptional gene regulation has become increasingly recognized.

Promoter hypermethylation – induced inactivation of tumor suppressor genes is an important mechanism that leads to gastric carcinogenesis. For example, CDH1, the gene encoding epithelial cadherin (E – cadherin), is a tumor suppressor gene located on chromosome 16q22. 1. E – cadherin is expressed in normal epithelium and plays a role in calcium – dependent cell adhesion. CDH1 is hypermethylated in 40% to 80% of human primary gastric carcinoma. In diffuse gastric cancer, a methylation – induced decrease in E – cadherin expression has been observed in more than 50% of the undifferentiated early cancers and adjacent non – cancerous gastric epithelial tissues. Therefore, CDH1 methylation – induced loss of E – cadherin expression is an early event in the malignant transformation of gastric mucosa. E – cadherin is also inactivated by mutation and accounts for the hereditary nature of diffuse – type gastric cancer. Runt – related transcription factor 3 (RUNX3) is a key molecule in the transforming growth factor – β (TGF – β) signaling pathway. The expression of RUNX3 is significantly reduced in gastric cancer. The main reason for the decreased RUNX3 expression is DNA hypermethylation in the promoter region. Kim et al. found that RUNX3 CpG island methylation occurs in 8. 1% of chronic gastritis cases, 28. 1% of intestinal metaplasia cases,

27.3% of gastric adenocarcinoma cases, 64% of primary gastric
cancer cases and 60% of gastric cancer cell lines. In RUNX3 knock-
out mice, apoptosis is inhibited. These mice show hypertrophy of gastric mucosa and intestinal metaplasia of gastric epithelial cells, indicating that RUNX3 hypermethylation plays an important role in the
malignant transformation of intestinal – type gastric cancer. Additionally, chronic gastritis, intestinal metaplasia, gastric adenoma and gastric cancer show an increasing frequency of p16/cyclin – dependent
kinase inhibitor 2A (CDKN2A) methylation. This finding indicates
that p16/CDKN2A methylation occurs at the initial stage of gastric
mucosal malignant transformation and undergoes cumulative change as
the disease progresses. Genes related to the malignant transformation
of gastric mucosa that undergo promoter methylation also include the
retinoblastoma (RB) gene, von Hippel – Lindau (VHL) tumor suppressor gene, breast cancer 1 (BRCA1) gene, human mutL homolog
1 (hMLH1) gene, X – ray repair cross – complementationgroup
1 (XRCC1) gene and ADAM metallopeptidase with thrombospondin
type 1 motif 9 (ADAMTS9) gene.

In gastric cancer, the distribution characteristics of gene methylation are correlated with biological tumor characteristics and patient
prognosis. Patrick Tan and colleagues investigated DNA methylation
profiles of 240 primary gastric cancers and gastric cancer cell lines. It
has been found that methylomes are widely distributed in gastric cancers. However, these results need to be further verified. In addition,
previous data on the methylation of gastric mucosal transformation –
related genes are mainly derived from experimental studies of previously established cell lines or small – sized clinical tissue specimen
studies. The current knowledge on gene methylation is far from being

accurate and comprehensive. Future studies focusing on the following aspects will be more valuable: 1. Longitudinal studies: large – scale DNA methylation profiling of clinical tissue specimens – Longitudinal, dynamic cohort studies that analyze serial clinical specimens obtained from individual patients at various stages, from inflammation, intestinal metaplasia, and atypical hyperplasia to gastric cancer, are particularly inadequate; a genome – wide longitudinal study of DNA methylation based on such specimens will provide more accurate and comprehensive results; 2. Data mining: collection and analysis of the data on gene methylation in normal gastric mucosa, precancerous lesions and gastric cancer in various populations – Exploration of the methylation pattern changes that occur during the malignant transformation of gastric mucosa using large – scale data mining allows a complete understanding of the gene methylation characteristics related to the malignant transformation of gastric mucosa as well as the differentiation of the key methylation changes from the numerous accompanying changes. 3. Non – CpG methylation: non – CpG methylationis an emerging field of research. However, few data have been obtained for gastric cancer. The research on the distribution, recognition and regulation of non – CpG methylation in gastric cancer will further deepen our understanding of epigenetic regulation in the transformation of gastric mucosa.

The histone code affects the malignant transformation of gastric mucosa

In eukaryotes, DNA, histones and nonhistone proteins are arranged in a highly ordered pattern to form chromatin. Histones are divided into 5 classes, including nucleosomal core histones (H2A, H2B, H3 and H4) and linker histones (H1). Each core histone consists of a globular structural domain and an N – terminal tail that is exposed on the surface of the nucleosome. A variety of covalent modifications may occur at the N – terminus of the core histones, including acetylation, methylation, phosphorylation, ubiquitination and glycosylation. These histone modifications alter the chromatin structure and therefore determine the state of gene activation/inactivation; these modifications also regulate physiological processes in the cells. Different histone modifications are orchestrated in both time and space, forming a complex regulatory network known as the "histone code". Numerous studies have demonstrated histone modification changes in gastric cancer, and such changes are of great clinical significance. Recent studies of gastric cancer – related histone modifications have mainly focused on histone acetylation, methylation and phosphorylation.

Histone acetylation: Histone acetylation is co – regulated by histoneacetyltransferases (HATs) and histone deacetylases (HDACs). Histone acetylation promotes transcription, whereas histone deacetylation inhibits transcription. Abnormal expression of HDACs and HATs is frequently observed in gastric precancerous lesions and gastric cancer. Current studies have found that histone deacetylation occurs at the promoter region of a number of genes in gastric cancer, including p21 (WAF1/CIP1), RIP – associated ICH1/CED3 – homologous protein with a death domain (RAIDD), DTW domain containing 1 (DTWD1), p53 upregulated modulator of apoptosis (PUMA), gelsolin and retinoic acid receptor beta, deleted in liver cancer – 1 (DLC1) and thioredoxin – interacting protein (TXNIP). In addition, histone deacetylation has been shown to be positively correlated with the downregulated expression of the above genes.

Histone methylation: Histone methylation mainly occurs at the lysine (K) and arginine (R) residuesof H3 and H4 and is regulated by histone methyltransferases (HMTs) and histone demethylases (HDMs). There are 3 types of histone methylation: monomethylation, dimethylation and trimethylation. Different sites and types of histone methylation confer-different functions. Methylation of H3K9 and H4K20 inhibits gene expression, whereas methylation of H3K4, H3K36 and H3K79 activates gene expression. H3K27 monomethylation activates gene expression, whereas H3K27 dimethylation and trimethylation inhibit gene expression. For example, H3K27 trimethylation inhibits the expression of Arg kinase – binding protein 2 (ArgBP2) in gastric cancer.

Histone phosphorylation: Phosphorylation can disrupt the interaction between histones and DNA and renders the chromatin structure unstable. In addition, phosphorylation may create a surface that binds to protein recognition modules, thereby allowing interaction with specific protein complexes. These two mechanisms enable histone phosphorylation to play a role in chromosome condensation/separation, transcription activation, apoptosis and DNA damage repair. Studies on the role of histone phosphorylation in the malignant transformation of gastric mucosa are insufficient. Fehri et al. found that H. pylori infection reduces the phosphorylation levels of histone H3S10 and H3T3 in gastric epithelial cells, thus regulating the cell cycle. This finding may represent an important mechanism of H. pylori – induced gastric carcinogenesis. In addition, an increased phosphorylation level of histone H3 was shown to be closely related to the histological type, vascular infiltration and lymph node metastasis of gastric cancer and is an independent factor associated with a poor prognosis in patients with gastric cancer. The findings indirectly support the hypothesis that histone phosphorylation is involved in the malignant transformation of gastric mucosal cells.

However, relevant studies remain focused on the relationships between the changes in the overall level of certain histone modifications and various pathological states during gastric mucosal carcinogenesis. Studies investigating the mechanisms through which histone modifications affect the malignant transformation of gastric mucosa are currently lacking. To pinpoint the genes or signaling pathways through which histone modifications affect the malignant transformation of gastric mucosa, studies that utilize histone modification – specific antibodies to coprecipitate chromatin or those that employ oligonucleotide microarrays or deep DNA sequencing to identify significantly differentially modified gene loci/chromatin segments and then combine these discoveries with gene function verification would be beneficial.

Non – coding RNAs regulate the malignant transformation of gastric mucosal epithelial cells

Non – coding RNAs (ncRNAs) is a general term for an RNA molecule that does not encode a protein. NcRNAs include micro RNA (miRNA), piwi – interacting RNA (piRNA), long non – coding RNA (lncRNA), transfer RNA (tRNA) and ribosomal RNA (rRNA). A large number of studies have focused on the roles of miRNAs and lncRNAs in gastric carcinogenesis.

miRNA

miRNAs are a class of evolutionarily conserved, endogenous, non – protein – coding small RNAs. miRNAs participate in the malignant transformation of gastric mucosal cells by negatively regulating the expression of target genes.

Abnormal expression of miRNA molecules in gastric cancer.
Petrocca et al. compared the miRNA expression profiles between tissues with histological signs of chronic gastritis and normal gastric mucosa. It has been found that, in chronic gastritis, the expression of miR – 1 and miR – 155 is upregulated whereas the expression of miR – 20, miR – 26b, miR – 202, miR – 203 and miR – 205 is downregulated. Ueda et al. examined miRNA expression in 160 paired samples of gastric cancer tissues and non – cancerous tissues. The authors found that the expression of 22 miRNAs is upregulated while the expression of 13 miRNAs is downregulated in gastric cancer tissues compared with the non – cancerous tissues. In addition, 83% of the patients with gastric cancer could be accurately diagnosed based on miRNA expression profiles in tissue specimens. Microarrayanalysis has been performed to examine miRNA expression in gastric cancer tissue specimens collected in a large number of countries and geographical regions. The results have shown that the expression of miR – 21, miR – 27aand miR – 196a is significantly elevated in gastric cancer, whereas the expression of lethal – 7 (let – 7) miRNA, miR – 101 and miR – 29a is markedly reduced. These results clearly demonstrate that miRNAs are involved in gastric carcinogenesis. However, the consistency of previous results is poor. This may be due to sample variation. At present, there is no generally accepted characteristic miRNA expression profile of gastric cancer. Further studies of large and multicenter sample cohort(s) are needed.

Abnormal expression of miRNAs significantly affects the malignant phenotype of gastric cancer cells. The expression of miR – 847 is decreased in gastric cancer, which activates the signal transducer and activator of transcription 3 (STAT3)/vascular endothelial growth factor A (VEGF – A) pathway, increases tumor angiogenesis and promotes the development and progression of gastric cancer. The expression of miR – 145 is upregulated in gastric cancer, which inhibits the expression of catenin (cadherin – associated protein), delta 1 (CTNND1) and N – cadherin while promoting the translocation of CTNND1 and E – cadherin from the cytoplasm to the cell membrane. As a result, the proliferation and metastasis of gastric cancer cells are promoted, and the apoptosis of gastric cancer cells is inhibited. The expression of the miR – 106b – 25 cluster is upregulated in gastric cancer, which inhibits the TGF – β pathway, induces the downregulation of the expression of cyclin – dependent kinase inhibitor 1A (CDKN1A) and BCL2 – like 11 apoptosis facilitator (BCL2L11), and promotes the development and progression of gastric cancer. Our study demonstrated that the expression of miR – 17 – 5p is significantly increased in gastric cancer tissues. High miR – 17 – 5p expression inhibits suppressor of cytokine signaling 6(SOCS6), which promotes the proliferation of gastric cancer cells . The expression of miR – 296 – 5p is abnormally increased in gastric cancer, which inhibits the expression of caudal – related homeobox 1 (CDX1). Furthermore, miR – 296 – 5p/ CDX1 affects the phosphorylation level of the extracellular signal – regulated kinases 1 and 2 (ERK1/2) through the mitogen – activated protein kinase (MAPK)/ERK pathway and induces changes in the expression levels of the cell cycle – related protein cyclin D1 and the apoptosis – related proteins B – cell lymphoma 2 (Bcl2) and BCL2 – associated X (Bax), thus maintaining the survival of gastric cancer cells and regulating cell proliferation, miR – 149, miR – 7, miR – 199a – 5p, miR – 206, miR – 19a/b and miR – 218 are all involved in the development and progression of gastric cancer.

lncRNA

LncRNA refers to a class of RNA molecules greater than 200 nucleotides (nt) in length, that are transcribed mainly by RNA polymerase II, that lack apparent open reading frames (ORFs) and that do not encode proteins. However, lncRNAs participate in the regulation of a variety of intracellular signaling processes (including tumorigenesis) through the modification of chromatins, activation of transcription and interference with transcription. Recent studies have shown that several lncRNAs are abnormally expressed in gastric cancer. Moreover, abnormal expression of lncRNAs plays an important role in the development, progression, invasion and metastasis of gastric cancer.

HOXtranscriptantisense intergenic RNA (HOTAIR) is located on chromosome 12q13. 13. HOTAIR is a 2158 − nt lncRNA that possesses a trans − regulatory function. The 5′ end of HOTAIR binds to the initiation complex known as polycomb repressive complex 2 (PRC2). Binding of HOTAIR to PRC2 induces the phosphorylation of EZH2, a subunit of PRC2, at threonine 345 and the subsequent trimethylation of chromosome − bound histone H3K27, thereby inhibiting the expression of the target genes. In addition, the 3′ end of HOTAIR binds to the lysine − specific demethylase 1 (LSD1)/RESTcorepressor 1 (CoREST)/repressor element 1 (RE1) silencing transcription factor (REST) complex, which mediates histone H3K4me2 demethylation and thereby regulates the transcriptional activity of target genes. HOTAIR expression is significantly increased in gastric cancer tissues compared with paracancerous tissues. In diffuse gastric cancer, the high HOTAIR expression group exhibits drastically increased invasion and lymph node metastasis and a decreased overall survival rate in comparison to the low HOTAIR expression group. In addition, studies have shown that inhibition of HOTAIR expression in gastric cancer cells decreases the expression of matrix metalloproteinases 1 and 3, reduces the invasive capability of cancer cells and reverses the epithelial – mesenchymal transition (EMT) in gastric cancer cells. These findings demonstrate that HOTAIR plays an important role in the development and progression of gastric cancer. The H19 gene (full – length: 2.5 kb) is located on the human chromosome 11p15.5 region and contains a total of 5 exons and 4 introns. The processed, mature H19 has a length of 2.3 kb. Due to the lack of obvious ORFs, H19 is defined as an lncRNA. H19 expression is significantly elevated in gastric cancer tissues compared to paracancerous tissues. Overexpression of H19 enhances the proliferative capacity of the cells, whereas small interfering RNA (siRNA) – mediated interference of H19 expression enhances apoptosis. The effects of overexpression and downregulation of H19 are related to the inactivation and activation of the TP53 gene. Recent studies have shown that transcription of the H19 gene also produces a mature miRNA, namely miR –675. H19 is capable of regulating the progression of gastric cancer through the H19/miR – 675/runt – related transcription factor 1 (RUNX1) signaling axis. In addition, tumor suppressor candidate 7 (TUSC7), maternally expressed 3 (MEG3), BM742401, colon cancer associated transcript 1 (CCAT1) and multidrug resistant (MDR) – related and upregulatedlncRNA (MRUL) have been found to be differentially expressed between gastric cancer cells and normal gastric mucosal cells and affect the malignant phenotype of gastric cancer cells.

　　Current studies in the field of ncRNAs have mainly focused on the effects of such molecules on the malignant phenotypes of gastric cancer cells including growth, proliferation, metastasis and drug resistance. The conclusion that ncRNAs participate in the malignant transformation of gastric mucosal cells is based on the findings that ncRNAs are differentially expressed between normal gastric mucosal cells and gastric cancer cells and that the differential expression of ncRNAs induces functional changes in certain malignant phenotype of gastric cancer cells. There are virtually no functional studies that directly address the malignant transformation of normal gastric mucosa. In addition, the intrinsic link between various ncRNA molecules remains unclear. We simulated the interactions between a number of gastric carcinogenesis – related molecules that have been identified by our study or reported in the literature (Figure 1). However, further biological experiments are required to discover the ncRNA regulated network.

H. pylori infection promotes gastric cancer mainly through epigenetic regulation

H. pyloriinfection is the most important risk factor for gastric cancer. The epigenetic changes induced by H. pylori compose one of the principal molecular mechanisms of gastric carcinogenesis.

H. pyloriinfection and gene methylation. Numerous studies have demonstrated that H. pylori infection is closely related to abnormal CpG island methylation. Maekita et al. found that methylation levels of all the detected regions were much higher in H. pylori – positive samples than in H. pylori – negative samples among healthy volunteers. Nakajima et al. analyzed the promoter methylation of CpG islands of 48 genes that may be methylated in gastric cancer cell lines. The results showed that 26 genes were consistently methylated in individuals with current or past infection by H. pylori. Shin et al. i-

dentified quite distinct methylation profiles according to the presence
or absence of current H. pylori infection in non – cancerous gastric
mucosae from patients with gastric cancer. Cheng concluded that
FOXD3 – mediated transcriptional control of tumor suppressors is de-
regulated by H. pylori infection – induced hypermethylation. This in
turn could affect the suppression of gastric tumors. These findings in-
dicate that H. pylori infection potently induces CpG island methylation
and may be responsible for the initiation of gastric carcinogenesis.

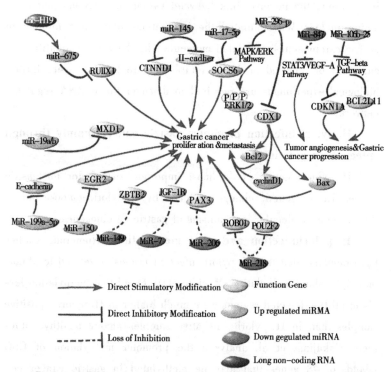

Figure 1　ncRNA – oriented network in the malignant transformation process of gastric
cancer. This figure provides insight into the roles of ncRNA and its related protein in the
malignant transformation of gastric mucosal cells. It can be seen that a complex networkcom-
posed of ncRNA and its upstream and downstream componentsaffects the malignant transformation of gastric mucosal cells

H. pylori – mediated chronic inflammation is one of the important causes of DNA methylation. A number of studies have suggested that methylation levels in the gastric mucosa after H. pylori infection decrease after H. pylori eradication. These data support the idea that H. pylori – mediated inflammation induces methylation. However, how the inflammation triggers DNA methylation is not yet known.

H. pylori infection and histone modification.

Relatively few studies have investigated whether Helicobacter pylori affects histone modifications. The infection of gastric epithelial cells with H. pylori leads to hyperacetylation of histone H4, which induces the binding of histone H1 to ATP and causes histone H3 dephosphorylation and deacetylation. These changes result in the abnormal expression of oncogenes and tumor suppressor genes, which contributes to malignant transformation of gastric epithelial cells.

H. pylori infection is a major cause of abnormal miRNA expression. MiRNAs play an important role in H. pylori infection – induced malignant transformation of gastric mucosa. Zhang et al. demonstrated for the first time that H. pylori infection is able to induce changes in miRNA expression profiles. They found that miR – 21 expression is significantly increased in H. pylori – positive gastric tissues, indicating that the increased expression of miR – 21 may be related to H. pylori infection. In AGS human gastric carcinoma cells, H. pylori infection promotes the secretion of nuclear factor kappa B (NF – κB) and interleukin 6 (IL – 6) and activates activator protein 1 (AP – 1) and STAT3, resulting in significantly upregulated miR – 21 expression and drastically enhanced cell proliferative and invasive capabilities. Using miRNA microarrays, Matsushima et al. identified 55 miRNAs that were differentially expressed between H. pylori – positive and H. pylori – negative endoscopic biopsy specimens. Among the 55 miR-NAs, the expression of 30 miRNAs was significantly reduced. A portion of the miRNAs (including miR – 223, miR – 375 and miR – 200c) were found to be significantly correlated with gastric mucosal inflammatory activity, chronic inflammation and H. pylori infection severity scores. Correlation analysis showed that 8 miRNAs can be used to accurately predict whether H. pylori infection is present. Infection of the cells with an H. pylori strain containing the wild – type CagA (cytotoxin – associated gene A) structural domain induced changes in the expression of certain miRNAs (e. g. , let – 7, miR – 125a and miR – 500) , whereas H. pylori strains with mutant CagA showed no such effect. Studies conducted by Saito et al. showed that miR – 17 and miR – 20a are also involved in the gastric cancer – promoting signaling pathways mediated by CagA. CagA activates c – Myc through the activation of the Erk pathway, which further stimulates the expression of miR – 17 and miR – 20a. MiR – 20a is capable of suppressing p21 expression. In addition, miR – 146a, miR – 155 and miR – 218 are also involved in H. pylori infection – related malignant transformation of gastric mucosa. In a study conducted by Matsushima et al. , patients who tested positive for H. pylori infection were successfully cured with an anti – H. pylori regimen and were re – examined 4 weeks after eradication of H. pylori infection. Cure of the H. pylori infection not only restored the levels of 14 miRNAs whose expression was downregulated during H. pylori infection but also significantly reduced the levels of a portion of the miRNAs whose expression was upregulated by H. pylori infection. This phenomenon indicates that downregulation/inhibition of the expression of cancer – promoting miRNAs using methods such as oligonucleotides and miRNA sponges combined with the introduction of exogenous cancer – suppressing miRNAs may reduce or even partially block the promoting effect of H. pylori on gastric cancer.

The effects of various types of epigenetic regulations (such as DNAmethylation, histone modificationand ncRNA) on the malignant transformation of gastric mucosaare not independent. Instead, the epigenetic effects interact synergistically to promotegastric carcinogenesis. Additionally, different epigenetic changes may coordinate in the regulation of the expression of one carcinogenesis – related gene (Figure 2). For example,ubiquitin – like containing PHD and RING finger domains 1 (UHRF1) is known to maintain DNA methylation via the recruitment of DNA methyltransferase1 (DNMT1). We identified and verifiedmiR – 146a/b as direct upstream regulators of UHRF1. Duursma et al. found that miR – 148 targets human DNMT3b. miR – 146a/b and miR – 148 can regulate RUNX3 expression via the effects of UHRF1 and DNMT1 on promoter methylation. In addition, increased H3K9 dimethylation and reduced H3 acetylation synergistically inhibit the transcription of RUNX3. Moreover, miR – 130b, miR – 301a, miR, miR – 103a, miR – 495,and miR – 532 – 5p directly inhibit RUNX3 translation at the post – transcriptional level. Decreased RUNX3 expression directly downregulates miR – 30a expression, which enhances the expression of the miR – 30a target gene vimentin and promotes EMT in gastric cancercells. RUNX3 regulates gastric cancer cell proliferation via the TGF – β and Wnt pathways and affects angiogenesis in gastric cancer by regulating the expression of vascular endothelial growth factor (VEGF). In contrast, different epigenetic changes may regulate the expression of different carcinogenesis –

related genes, whereby they cooperate to promote the malignant transformation of gastric mucosa.

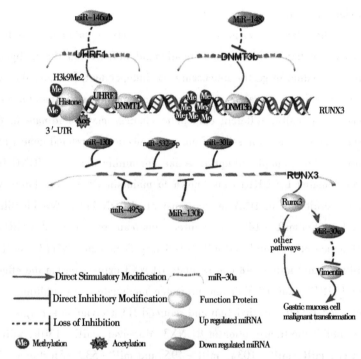

Figure 2   Epigenetic regulation of RUNX3 in the malignant transformation of gastric mucosal cells. MiR – 146a/b and miR – 148 directly inhibited UHRF1 and DNMT3b, respectively. Downregulation of miR – 146a/b and miR – 148 led to the increase in UHRF1 and DNMT3b, and this effect in turn inactivated RUNX3 via promoter methylation in gastric cancer. Additionally, increased H3K9 dimethylation and reduced H3 acetylation, as well as the increasedmiR – 130b, miR – 301a, miR – 106a, miR – 103a, miR – 495, and miR – 532 – 5p, synergistically inhibitedthe expression of RUNX3

Conclusions

The exploitation of characteristic epigenetic alterations during the malignant transformation of gastric mucosa allows for the prevention, diagnosis, treatmentand prognostic evaluation of gastric cancer from a new perspective independent of protein expression. For example, it has been reported that promoter methylation of death – associated protein kinase (DAPK), E – cadherin and p16 genes may serve as a criterion forsensitive and specific diagnosis of gastric cancer. We have found that the methylation status of the ring finger protein 180 (RNF180) gene may be used topredict the malignant potential of intestinal metaplasia and atypical hyperplasia of gastric mucosa and diagnose early gastric cancer (unpublished data). Currently, we have established a fluorescence – based quantitative technique that enables the analysis of RNF180gene methylation and meets the registration requirements for diagnostic reagents. We have initiated aclinical trial applicationto test this diagnostic kit.

The reversibility of epigenetic alterations (such as DNA methylation and histone modification) has recently become a hot topic in drug development. Studies have found that inhibition of deacetylase may suppress the malignant phenotype of gastric cancer cells and increase the sensitivity of gastric cancer cells to chemotherapy. Histone deacetylase inhibitors such as Vorinostat (Zolinza, suberoylanilide hydroxamic acid, SAHA) developed by Merck & Co., Inc. (USA) and Chidamide developed in China have been successfully used in the

clinical treatment of cancer. Currently, a number of DNA methyltransferase inhibitors (DNMTi) and histone deacetylase inhibitors are undergoing clinical trials to assess their safety and efficacy for the treatment of tumors.

However, unfavorable epigenetic changes induced by epigenetic
drugs may lead to severe side effects. The discovery of ways by which
the specificity against tumor cells can be enhanced and the side
effects can be reduced is still a hot topic. The epigenetic modifications
and their combinations that are involved in the malignant transformation of gastric mucosa are highly complex and diverse. There are many
outstanding issues requiring clarification. In – depth studies and further elucidation of the epigenetic networks that regulate the malignant
transformation of gastric mucosa will provide a wealth of pathways and
targets for understanding gastric cancer development and progression,
conducting molecular typing, establishing new therapies and developing new drugs.

Acknowledgments

Our research is supported by the National Science Foundation of
China (NO. 81272649, NO. 81430072, NO. 81272203).

（帖　君　张向远　樊代明）

Reference

[1] Torre LA, Bray F, Siegel RL, et al. Global cancer statistics. CA Cancer J Clin,. 2012,65 (2):87 – 108. DOI:10. 3322/caac. 21262.

[2] Chen W. Cancer statistics: updated cancer burden in China. Chinese journal of cancer research, 2015, 27 (1):1. DOI: 10. 3978/j. issn. 1000 – 9604. 2015. 02. 07.

[3] Wang K, Kan J, Yuen ST, et al. Exome sequencing identifies frequent mutation of ARID1A in molecular subtypes of gastric cancer. Nat Genet, 2011, 43 (12):1219 – 1223. DOI:10. 1038/ng. 982.

[4] Liang Q, Yao X, Tang S, et al. Integrative identification of Epstein – Barr virus – associated mutations and epigenetic alterations in gastric cancer. Gastroenterology. 2014, 147 (6): 1350 – 1362, e1354. DOI: 10. 1053/j. gastro. 2014. 08. 036.

[5] Waddington CH. Preliminary Notes on the Development of the Wings in Normal and Mutant Strains of Drosophila. Proc Natl Acad Sci USA, 1939, 25 (7):299 – 307.

[6] Dobrilla G, Benvenuti S, Amplatz S, et al. Chronic gastritis, intestinal metaplasia, dysplasia and Helicobacter pylori in gastric cancer: putting the pieces together. The Italian journal of gastroenterology, 1994, 26 (9): 449 – 458.

[7] Correa P. Helicobacter pylori and gastric carcinogenesis. The American journal of surgical pathology, 1995, 19(1):S37 – 43.

[8] Gigek CO, Chen ES, Calcagno DQ, et al. Epigenetic mechanisms in gastric cancer. Epigenomics, 2012, 4 (3):279 – 294. DOI:10. 2217/epi. 12. 22.

[9] Calcagno DQ, de Arruda Cardoso Smith M, Burbano RR. Cancer type – specific epigenetic changes: gastric cancer. Methods Mol Biol, 2015, 1238:79 – 101.

DOI:10. 1007/978 – 1 – 4939 – 1804 – 1_5.

[10] Bird AP. CpG – rich islands and the function of DNA methylation. Nature, 1986,321 (6067):209 – 213. DOI:10. 1038/321209a0.

[11] Aran D, Hellman A. DNA methylation of transcriptional enhancers and cancer predisposition. Cell, 2013, 154 (1):11 – 13. DOI: 10. 1016/j. cell. 2013. 06. 018.

[12] Grady WM, Willis J, Guilford PJ, et al. Methylation of the CDH1 promoter as the second genetic hit in hereditary diffuse gastric cancer. Nat Genet, 2000,26 (1):16 – 17. DOI:10. 1038/79120.

[13] Chan AO, Lam SK, Wong BC, et al. Promoter methylation of E – cadherin gene in gastric mucosa associated with Helicobacter pylori infection and in gastric cancer. Gut,2003,52 (4):502 – 506.

[14] Kim TY, Lee HJ, Hwang KS, et al. Methylation of RUNX3 in various types of human cancers and premalignant stages of gastric carcinoma. Lab Invest,2004,84 (4):479 – 484. DOI:10. 1038/labinvest. 3700060.

[15] Sato F, Meltzer SJ. CpG island hypermethylation in progression of esophageal and gastric cancer. Cancer,2006,106(3):483 – 493. DOI:10. 1002/cncr. 21657.

[16] Lu XX, Yu JL, Ying LS, et al. Stepwise cumulation of RUNX3 methylation mediated by Helicobacter pylori infection contributes to gastric carcinoma progression. Cancer, 2012, 118 (22): 5507 – 5517. DOI: 10. 1002/cncr. 27604.

[17] Lu ZM, Zhou J, Wang X, et al. Nucleosomes correlate with in vivo progression pattern of de novo methylation of p16 CpG islands in human gastric carcinogenesis. PLoS One,2012,7 (4):e35928. DOI:10. 1371/journal. pone. 0035928.

[18] Kang GH, Lee S, Kim JS, et al. Profile of aberrant CpG island methylation along the multistep pathway of gastric carcinogenesis. Lab Invest,2003,83 (5):635 – 641.

[19] Kang GH, Lee S, Kim JS, et al. Profile of aberrant CpG island methylation along multistep gastric carcinogenesis. Lab Invest, 2003, 83 (4): 519 – 526.

[20] Kim H, Kim YH, Kim SE, et al. Concerted promoter hypermethylation of hMLH1, p16INK4A, and E – cadherin in gastric carcinomas with microsatellite instability. J Pathol, 2003, 200 (1): 23 – 31. DOI: 10. 1002/path. 1325.

[21] Tahara T, Arisawa T. DNA methylation as a molecular biomarker in gastric cancer. Epigenomics, 2015, 7 (3): 475 – 486. DOI: 10. 2217/epi. 15. 4.

[22] Zouridis H, Deng N, Ivanova T, et al. Methylation subtypes and large – scale epigenetic alterations in gastric cancer. Sci Transl Med, 2012, 4 (156): 6721 – 6727. DOI: 10. 1126/scitranslmed. 3004504.

[23] Berger SL. Molecular biology: The histone modification circus. Science, 2001, 292 (5514): 64 – 65.

[24] Yang Y, Yin X, Yang H, et al. Histone demethylase LSD2 acts as an E3 ubiquitin ligase and inhibits cancer cell growth through promoting proteasomal degradation of OGT. Mol Cell, 2015, 58 (1): 47 – 59. DOI: 10. 1016/j. molcel. 2015. 01. 038.

[25] Song J, Noh JH, Lee JH, et al. Increased expression of histone deacetylase 2 is found in human gastric cancer. APMIS, 2005, 113 (4): 264 – 268. DOI: 10. 1111/j. 1600 – 0463. 2005. apm_04. x.

[26] Sudo T, Mimori K, Nishida N, et al. Histone deacetylase 1 expression in gastric cancer. Oncol Rep, 2011, 26 (4): 777 – 782. DOI: 10. 3892/or. 2011. 1361.

[27] Mitani Y, Oue N, Hamai Y, et al. Histone H3 acetylation is associated with reduced p21 (WAF1/CIP1) expression by gastric carcinoma. J Pathol, 2005, 205 (1): 65 – 73. DOI: 10. 1002/path. 1684.

[28] Shen Q, Tang W, Sun J, et al. Regulation of CRADD – caspase 2 cascade by histone deacetylase 1 in gastric cancer. Am J Transl Res, 2014, 6 (5):

538 - 547.

[29]　Ma Y,Yue Y,Pan M,et al. Histone deacetylase 3 inhibits new tumor suppressor gene DTWD1 in gastric cancer. American journal of cancer research,2015,5 (2):663 - 673.

[30]　Kim JH,Choi YK,Kwon HJ,et al. Downregulation of gelsolin and retinoic acid receptor beta expression in gastric cancer tissues through histone deacetylase 1. J Gastroenterol Hepatol,2004,19 (2):218 - 224.

[31]　Kim TY,Kim IS,Jong HS,et al. Transcriptional induction of DLC - 1 gene through Sp1 sites by histone deacetylase inhibitors in gastric cancer cells. Exp Mol Med,2008,40 (6):639 - 646. DOI:10. 3858/emm. 2008. 40. 6. 639.

[32]　Lee JH,Jeong EG,Choi MC,et al. Inhibition of histone deacetylase 10 induces thioredoxin - interacting protein and causes accumulation of reactive oxygen species in SNU - 620 human gastric cancer cells. Mol Cells,2010, 30 (2):107 - 112. DOI:10. 1007/s10059 - 010 - 0094 - z.

[33]　Tong Y, Li Y, Gu H, et al. MORC2 downregulates ArgBP2 via histone methylation in gastric cancer cells. Biochem Biophys Res Commun,2015. DOI:10. 1016/j. bbrc. 2015. 10. 059.

[34]　Fehri LF, Rechner C, Janssen S, et al. Helicobacter pylori - induced modification of the histone H3 phosphorylation status in gastric epithelial cells reflects its impact on cell cycle regulation. Epigenetics,2009,4 (8): 577 - 586.

[35]　Takahashi H,Murai Y,Tsuneyama K,et al. Overexpression of phosphorylated histone H3 is an indicator of poor prognosis in gastric adenocarcinoma patients. Appl Immunohistochem Mol Morphol,2006,14 (3):296 - 302.

[36]　Petrocca F,Visone R,Onelli MR,et al. E2F1 - regulated microRNAs impair TGFbeta - dependent cell - cycle arrest and apoptosis in gastric cancer. Cancer Cell, 2008, 13 (3):272 - 286. DOI:10. 1016/j. ccr. 2008. 02. 013.

[37] Ueda T,Volinia S,Okumura H,et al. Relation between microRNA expression and progression and prognosis of gastric cancer; a microRNA expression analysis. Lancet Oncol,2010,11 (2):136 – 146. DOI:10. 1016/S1470 – 2045(09)70343 – 2.

[38] Zhang Z,Li Z,Gao C,et al. miR – 21 plays a pivotal role in gastric cancer pathogenesis and progression. Lab Invest,2008,88 (12):1358 – 1366. DOI:10. 1038/labinvest. 2008. 94.

[39] Liu T,Tang H,Lang Y,et al. MicroRNA – 27a functions as an oncogene in gastric adenocarcinoma by targeting prohibitin. Cancer Lett,2009,273 (2):233 – 242. DOI:10. 1016/j. canlet. 2008. 08. 003.

[40] Sun M,Liu XH,Li JH,et al. MiR – 196a is upregulated in gastric cancer and promotes cell proliferation by downregulating p27(kip1). Mol Cancer Ther,2012,11 (4):842 – 852. DOI:10. 1158/1535 – 7163. MCT – 11 – 1015.

[41] Motoyama K,Inoue H,Nakamura Y,et al. Clinical significance of high mobility group A2 in human gastric cancer and its relationship to let – 7 microRNA family. Clin Cancer Res,2008,14(8):2334 – 2340. DOI:10. 1158/1078 – 0432. CCR – 07 – 4667.

[42] Zhou X,Xia Y,Li L,et al. MiR – 101 inhibits cell growth and tumorigenesis of Helicobacter pylori related gastric cancer by repression of SOCS2. Cancer Biol Ther,2015,16 (1):160 – 169. DOI:10. 4161/15384047. 2014. 987523.

[43] He XP,Shao Y,Li XL,et al. Downregulation of miR – 101 in gastric cancer correlates with cyclooxygenase – 2 overexpression and tumor growth. FEBS J,2012,279 (22):4201 – 4212. DOI:10. 1111/febs. 12013.

[44] Cui Y,Su WY,Xing J,et al. MiR – 29a inhibits cell proliferation and induces cell cycle arrest through the downregulation of p42. 3 in human gastric cancer. PLoS One,2011,6 (10):e25872. DOI:10. 1371/journal. pone. 0025872.

[45] Zhang X,Tang J,Zhi X,et al. miR – 874 functions as a tumor suppressor by inhibiting angiogenesis through STAT3/VEGF – A pathway in gastric cancer. Oncotarget,2015,6（3）:1605 – 1617. DOI:10. 18632/oncotarget. 2748.

[46] Xing AY,Wang YW,Su ZX,et al. Catenin – deltal,negatively regulated by miR – 145,promotes tumour aggressiveness in gastric cancer. J Pathol,2015,236（1）:53 –64. DOI:10. 1002/path. 4495.

[47] Wu Q,Luo G,Yang Z,et al. miR – 17 – 5p promotes proliferation by targeting SOCS6 in gastric cancer cells. FEBS Lett,2014,588（12）:2055 – 2062. DOI:10. 1016/j. febslet. 2014. 04. 036.

[48] Li T,Lu YY,Zhao XD,et al. MicroRNA – 296 – 5p increases proliferation in gastric cancer through repression of Caudal – related homeobox 1. Oncogene,2014,33（6）:783 – 793. DOI:10. 1038/onc. 2012. 637.

[49] Wu Q,Jin H,Yang Z,et al. MiR – 150 promotes gastric cancer proliferation by negatively regulating the pro – apoptotic gene EGR2. Biochem Biophys Res Commun,2010,392（3）:340 – 345. DOI:10. 1016/j. bbrc. 2009. 12. 182.

[50] Wang Y,Zheng X,Zhang Z,et al. MicroRNA – 149 inhibits proliferation and cell cycle progression through the targeting of ZBTB2 in human gastric cancer. PLoS One, 2012, 7（10）: e41693. DOI: 10. 1371/journal. pone. 0041693.

[51] Zhao X,Dou W,He L,et al. MicroRNA – 7 functions as an anti – metastatic microRNA in gastric cancer by targeting insulin – like growth factor – 1 receptor. Oncogene, 2013, 32（11）:1363 – 1372. DOI:10. 1038/onc. 2012. 156.

[52] Zhao X,He L,Li T,et al. SRF expedites metastasis and modulates the epithelial to mesenchymal transition by regulating miR – 199a – 5p expression in human gastric cancer. Cell Death Differ,2014,21（12）:1900 – 1913. DOI:10. 1038/cdd. 2014. 109.

[53] Zhang L,Xia L,Zhao L,et al. Activation of PAX3 - MET pathways due to miR - 206 loss promotes gastric cancer metastasis. Carcinogenesis,2015, 36 (3):390 - 399. DOI:10. 1093/carcin/bgv009.

[54] Zhang L,Liu X,Jin H,et al. miR - 206 inhibits gastric cancer proliferation in part by repressing cyclinD2. Cancer Lett,2013,332(1):94 - 101. DOI:10. 1016/j. canlet. 2013. 01. 023.

[55] Wu Q,Yang Z,Wang F,et al. MiR - 19b/20a/92a regulates the self - renewal and proliferation of gastric cancer stem cells. J Cell Sci,2013,126 (18):4220 - 4229. DOI:10. 1242/jcs. 127944.

[56] Tie J,Pan Y,Zhao L,et al. MiR - 218 inhibits invasion and metastasis of gastric cancer by targeting the Robo1 receptor. PLoS Genet,2010,6 (3): e1000879. DOI:10. 1371/journal. pgen. 1000879.

[57] Wang SM,Tie J,Wang WL,et al. POU2F2 - oriented network promotes human gastric cancer metastasis. Gut, 2015. DOI: 10. 1136/gutjnl - 2014 - 308932.

[58] Zhang Z,Li Z,Gao C,et al. miR - 21 plays a pivotal role in gastric cancer pathogenesis and progression. Lab Invest,2008. DOI:10. 1038/labinvest. 2008. 94.

[59] Matsushima K,Isomoto H,Inoue N,et al. MicroRNA signatures in Helicobacter pylori - infected gastric mucosa. Int J Cancer, 2011, 128 (2): 361 - 370. DOI:10. 1002/ijc. 25348.

[60] Saf C,Gulcan EM,Ozkan F,et al. Assessment of p21,p53 expression,and Ki - 67 proliferative activities in the gastric mucosa of children with Helicobacter pylori gastritis. Eur J Gastroenterol Hepatol,2015,27 (2):155 - 161. DOI:10. 1097/MEG. 0000000000000246.

[61] Saito Y,Murata - Kamiya N,Hirayama T,et al. Conversion of Helicobacter pylori CagA from senescence inducer to oncogenic driver through polarity - dependent regulation of p21. J Exp Med,2010,207 (10):2157 - 2174. DOI:10. 1084/jem. 20100602.

[62] Hayashi Y,Tsujii M,Wang J,et al. CagA mediates epigenetic regulation to attenuate let - 7 expression in Helicobacter pylori - related carcinogenesis. Gut, 2013,62(11):1536 - 1546. DOI:10. 1136/gutjnl - 2011 - 301625.

[63] Liu Z,Xiao B,Tang B,et al. Up - regulated microRNA - 146a negatively modulate Helicobacter pylori - induced inflammatory response in human gastric epithelial cells. Microbes and infection / Institut Pasteur,2010,12 (11):854 - 863. DOI:10. 1016/j. micinf. 2010. 06. 002.

[64] Crone SG,Jacobsen A,Federspiel B,et al. microRNA - 146a inhibits G protein - coupled receptor - mediated activation of NF - kappaB by targeting CARD10 and COPS8 in gastric cancer. Mol Cancer,2012,11:71. DOI:10. 1186/1476 - 4598 - 11 - 71.

[65] Gao C,Zhang Z,Liu W,et al. Reduced microRNA - 218 expression is associated with high nuclear factor kappa B activation in gastric cancer. Cancer,2010,116 (1):41 - 49. DOI:10. 1002/cncr. 24743.

[66] Endo H,Shiroki T,Nakagawa T,et al. Enhanced expression of long non - coding RNA HOTAIR is associated with the development of gastric cancer. PLoS One, 2013, 8 (10): e77070. DOI: 10. 1371/journal. pone. 0077070.

[67] Du M,Wang W,Jin H,et al. The association analysis of lncRNA HOTAIR genetic variants and gastric cancer risk in a Chinese population. Oncotarget,2015,6 (31):31255 - 31262. DOI:10. 18632/oncotarget. 5158.

[68] Xu ZY,Yu QM,Du YA,et al. Knockdown of long non - coding RNA HOTAIR suppresses tumor invasion and reverses epithelial - mesenchymal transition in gastric cancer. Int J Biol Sci,2013,9 (6):587 - 597. DOI: 10. 7150/ijbs. 6339.

[69] Yang F,Bi J,Xue X,et al. Up - regulated long non - coding RNA H19 contributes to proliferation of gastric cancer cells. FEBS J, 2012, 279 (17):3159 - 3165. DOI:10. 1111/j. 1742 - 4658. 2012. 08694. x.

[70] Zhuang M,Gao W,Xu J,et al. The long non - coding RNA H19 - derived

miR - 675 modulates human gastric cancer cell proliferation by targeting tumor suppressor RUNX1. Biochem Biophys Res Commun, 2014, 448 (3):315 - 322. DOI:10. 1016/j. bbrc. 2013. 12. 126.

[71] Li H, Yu B, Li J, et al. Overexpression of lncRNA H19 enhances carcinogenesis and metastasis of gastric cancer. Oncotarget, 2014, 5 (8):2318 - 2329. DOI:10. 18632/oncotarget. 1913.

[72] Qi P, Xu MD, Shen XH, et al. Reciprocal repression between TUSC7 and miR - 23b in gastric cancer. Int J Cancer, 2015, 137 (6):1269 - 1278. DOI:10. 1002/ijc. 29516.

[73] Sun M, Xia R, Jin F, et al. Downregulated long noncoding RNA MEG3 is associated with poor prognosis and promotes cell proliferation in gastric cancer. Tumour Biol, 2014, 35(2):1065 - 1073. DOI:10. 1007/s13277 - 013 - 1142 - z.

[74] Park SM, Park SJ, Kim HJ, et al. A known expressed sequence tag, BM742401, is a potent lincRNA inhibiting cancer metastasis. Exp Mol Med, 2013, 45:e31. DOI:10. 1038/emm. 2013. 59.

[75] Mizrahi I, Mazeh H, Grinbaum R, et al. Colon Cancer Associated Transcript - 1 (CCAT1) Expression in Adenocarcinoma of the Stomach. Journal of Cancer, 2015, 6(2):105 - 110. DOI:10. 7150/jca. 10568.

[76] Wang Y, Zhang D, Wu K, et al. Long noncoding RNA MRUL promotes ABCB1 expression in multidrug - resistant gastric cancer cell sublines. Mol Cell Biol, 2014, 34(17):3182 - 3193. DOI:10. 1128/MCB. 01580 - 13.

[77] Fujii S, Ito K, Ito Y, et al. Enhancer of zeste homologue 2 (EZH2) down - regulates RUNX3 by increasing histone H3 methylation. J Biol Chem, 2008, 283 (25): 17324 - 17332. DOI: 10. 1074/jbc. M800224200.

[78] Lee SH, Kim J, Kim WH, et al. Hypoxic silencing of tumor suppressor RUNX3 by histone modification in gastric cancer cells. Oncogene, 2009, 28 (2):184 - 194. DOI:10. 1038/onc. 2008. 377.

[79] Lai KW, Koh KX, Loh M, et al. MicroRNA – 130b regulates the tumour suppressor RUNX3 in gastric cancer. Eur J Cancer, 2010, 46(8): 1456 – 1463. DOI: 10. 1016/j. ejca. 2010. 01. 036.

[80] Wang M, Li C, Yu B, et al. Overexpressed miR – 301a promotes cell proliferation and invasion by targeting RUNX3 in gastric cancer. J Gastroenterol, 2013, 48 (9): 1023 – 1033. DOI: 10. 1007/s00535 – 012 – 0733 – 6.

[81] Zhang Y, Lu Q, Cai X. MicroRNA – 106a induces multidrug resistance in gastric cancer by targeting RUNX3. FEBS Lett, 2013, 587 (18): 3069 – 3075. DOI: 10. 1016/j. febslet. 2013. 06. 058.

[82] Jiang H, Yu WW, Wang LL, et al. miR – 130a acts as a potential diagnostic biomarker and promotes gastric cancer migration, invasion and proliferation by targeting RUNX3. Oncol Rep, 2015, 34(3): 1153 – 1161. DOI: 10. 3892/or. 2015. 4099.

[83] Lee SH, Jung YD, Choi YS, et al. Targeting of RUNX3 by miR – 130a and miR – 495 cooperatively increases cell proliferation and tumor angiogenesis in gastric cancer cells. Oncotarget, 2015, 6(32): 33269 – 33278. DOI: 10. 18632/oncotarget. 5037.

[84] Xu X, Zhang Y, Liu Z, et al. miRNA – 532 – 5p functions as an oncogenic microRNA in human gastric cancer by directly targeting RUNX3. J Cell Mol Med, 2016, 20 (1): 95 – 103. DOI: 10. 1111/jcmm. 12706.

[85] Liu Z, Chen L, Zhang X, et al. RUNX3 regulates vimentin expression via miR – 30a during epithelial – mesenchymal transition in gastric cancer cells. J Cell Mol Med, 2014, 18 (4): 610 – 623. DOI: 10. 1111/jcmm. 12209.

[86] Yano T, Ito K, Fukamachi H, et al. The RUNX3 tumor suppressor upregulates Bim in gastric epithelial cells undergoing transforming growth factor beta – induced apoptosis. Mol Cell Biol, 2006, 26 (12): 4474 – 4488. DOI: 10. 1128/MCB. 01926 – 05.

[87] Ito K. RUNX3 in oncogenic and anti – oncogenic signaling in gastrointesti-

nal cancers. J Cell Biochem,2011,112(5):1243 - 1249. DOI:10. 1002/jcb. 23047.

[88] Ito K,Lim AC,Salto - Tellez M,et al. RUNX3 attenuates beta - catenin/T cell factors in intestinal tumorigenesis. Cancer Cell,2008,14 (3):226 - 237. DOI:10. 1016/j. ccr. 2008. 08. 004.

[89] Peng Z,Wei D,Wang L,et al. RUNX3 inhibits the expression of vascular endothelial growth factor and reduces the angiogenesis,growth,and metastasis of human gastric cancer. Clin Cancer Res,2006,12(21):6386 - 6394. DOI:10. 1158/1078 - 0432. CCR - 05 - 2359.

[90] Kato K,Iida S,Uetake H,et al. Methylated TMS1 and DAPK genes predict prognosis and response to chemotherapy in gastric cancer. Int J Cancer,2008,122 (3):603 - 608. DOI:10. 1002/ijc. 23143.

[91] Xing X,Tang YB,Yuan G,et al. The prognostic value of E - cadherin in gastric cancer: a meta - analysis. Int J Cancer,2013,132 (11):2589 - 2596. DOI:10. 1002/ijc. 27947.

[92] Peng D,Zhang H,Sun G. The relationship between P16 gene promoter methylation and gastric cancer: a meta - analysis based on Chinese patients. Journal of cancer research and therapeutics,2014,10:292 - 295. DOI:10. 4103/0973 - 1482. 151535.

[93] Lee KH,Choi EY,Kim MK,et al. Inhibition of histone deacetylase activity down - regulates urokinase plasminogen activator and matrix metalloproteinase - 9 expression in gastric cancer. Mol Cell Biochem,2010,343(1 - 2):163 - 171. DOI:10. 1007/s11010 - 010 - 0510 - x.

[94] Lin L,Jiang H,Huang M,et al. Depletion of histone deacetylase 1 inhibits metastatic abilities of gastric cancer cells by regulating the miR - 34a/CD44 pathway. Oncol Rep,2015,34 (2):663 - 672. DOI:10. 3892/or. 2015. 4010.

[95] Regel I,Merkl L,Friedrich T,et al. Pan - histone deacetylase inhibitor panobinostat sensitizes gastric cancer cells to anthracyclines via induction

of CITED2. Gastroenterology,2012,143(1):99 – 109, e110. DOI:10. 1053/j. gastro. 2012. 03. 035.

[96] Song S,Wang Y,Xu P,et al. The inhibition of histone deacetylase 8 suppresses proliferation and inhibits apoptosis in gastric adenocarcinoma. Int J Oncol,2015. DOI:10. 3892/ijo. 2015. 3182.

[97] Yoon SN,Roh SA,Cho DH,et al. In vitro chemosensitivity of gastric adenocarcinomas to histone deacetylase inhibitors, compared to established drugs. Hepatogastroenterology,2010,57（99 – 100）:657 – 662.

[98] Zhang X,Yashiro M,Ren J,et al. Histone deacetylase inhibitor,trichostatin A,increases the chemosensitivity of anticancer drugs in gastric cancer cell lines. Oncol Rep,2006,16（3）:563 – 568.

[99] Li Y,Chen K,Zhou Y,et al. A New Strategy to Target Acute Myeloid Leukemia Stem and Progenitor Cells Using Chidamide,a Histone Deacetylase Inhibitor. Curr Cancer Drug Targets,2015,15（6）:493 – 503.

[100] Garcia – Manero G,Yang H,Bueso – Ramos C,et al. Phase 1 study of the histone deacetylase inhibitor vorinostat（suberoylanilide hydroxamic acid [SAHA]）in patients with advanced leukemias and myelodysplastic syndromes. Blood,2008,111（3）:1060 – 1066. DOI:10. 1182/blood – 2007 – 06 – 098061.

[101] Marks PA,Breslow R. Dimethyl sulfoxide to vorinostat:development of this histone deacetylase inhibitor as an anticancer drug. Nat Biotechnol, 2007,25（1）:84 – 90. DOI:10. 1038/nbt1272.

[102] McCarthy N. Epigenetics:Showing a more sensitive side. Nat Rev Cancer,2013,13（10）:680. DOI:10. 1038/nrc3605.

[103] Clozel T,Yang S,Elstrom RL,et al. Mechanism – based epigenetic chemosensitization therapy of diffuse large B – cell lymphoma. Cancer Discov,2013,3（9）:1002 – 1019. DOI:10. 1158/2159 – 8290. CD – 13 – 0117.

（原文已在线发表于 Cell Mol Life Sci,2016）

缩略词表

英文缩写	英文全称	中文全称
ADC	antibody – drug conjugate	抗体偶联药物
CAF	cancer – associated fibroblast	肿瘤相关成纤维细胞
CSF	colony stimulating factor	细胞集落刺激因子
Cyp	cyclophillin	亲环素
EMT	epithelial – mesenchymal transition	上皮间质转化
FUT	fucosyltransferase	岩藻糖转移酶
GGT	gamma – Glutamyl transpeptidese	伽玛谷氨酰转移酶
HIF	hypoxia inducible factor	缺氧诱导因子
Hp	Helicobacter pylori	幽门螺旋杆菌
HSP	heat shock protein	热休克蛋白
IGF	insulin – like growth factor	胰岛素样生长因子
IL	interleukin	白介素
MDR	multidrug resistence	多药耐药
MET	mesenchymal – epithelial transition	间充质上皮转化
MMP	matrix metalloproteinase	基质金属蛋白酶
PDX	patient – derived xenograft	患者来源的移植瘤模型
PSMA	prostate specific membrane antigen	前列腺特异性膜抗原
ROS	reactive oxygen species	活性氧物质
TAM	tumor – associated macrophage	肿瘤相关巨噬细胞
TNF	tumor necrosis factor	肿瘤坏死因子
VEGF	vascular endothelial growth factor	血管内皮生长因子